BENT

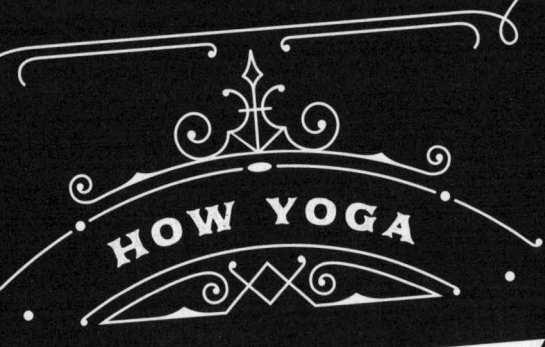

HOW YOGA

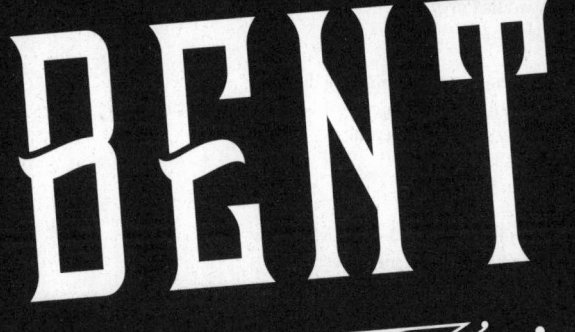

BENT

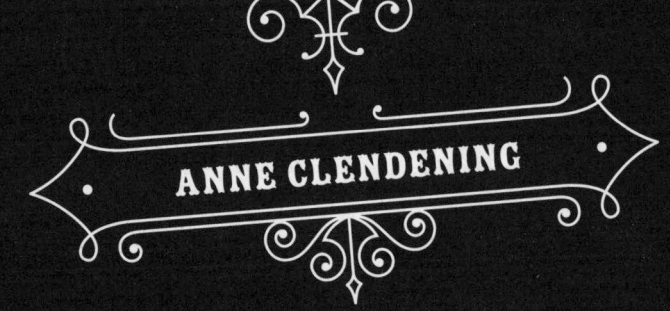

SAVED MY ASS

ANNE CLENDENING

PARALLAX
PRESS

BERKELEY, CALIFORNIA

Parallax Press
P.O. Box 7355
Berkeley, California 94707
www.parallax.org

Parallax Press is the publishing division
of Plum Village Community of Engaged Buddhism, Inc.
Printed in Canada

Cover and text design by Jess Morphew
Author photo © Gretchen Westlake
Illustrations © Vasya Kobelev / Shutterstock

ISBN: 978-1-941529-65-2

Library of Congress Cataloging-in-Publication Data

Names: Clendening, Anne, author.
Title: Bent : how yoga saved my ass / Anne Clendening.
Description: Berkeley, California : Parallax Press, 2019.
Identifiers: LCCN 2017023647 (print) | LCCN 2017048770 (ebook) | ISBN
   9781941529669 | ISBN 9781941529652
Subjects: LCSH: Clendening, Anne. | Spiritual biography. | Yoga.
Classification: LCC BL73.C54 (ebook) | LCC BL73.C54 A3 2019 (print) |
DDC
   613.7/046092 [B] --dc23
LC record available at https://lccn.loc.gov/201702364 7

1 2 3 4 5 / 21 20 19 18 17

For my parents

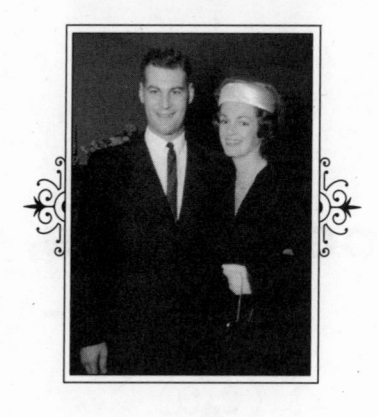

CONTENTS

INTRODUCTION

I'm sitting in a neurologist's office as sparsely decorated as a Saturday Night Live set. There's a desk with nothing on it, a swivel chair, and a long cushioned table with one of those loud strips of paper on it that I've never understood. They never even cover the whole thing.

The walls are another story. It seems whoever is in charge of the scenery has the same passion for laminated brain-disorder-centric wall hangings I once had for Leif Garrett posters. There's "Anatomy of the Brain," "Understanding Alzheimer's Disease: All You Need to Know About the Aging Brain, Dementia and Methods of Diagnosing A.D.," and a flow chart of "Immunological Markers in Neurological Disorders." I'm surprised there's not an actual human brain sitting around in a glass of formaldehyde.

Then again, nothing much would surprise me at this point.

Neurologist #3 is scribbling down notes on my "condition." I want to look, but I'm not sure if it's allowed. Instead I'm playing the commercial in my head with the guy cracking an egg into a frying pan. *This is your brain. This is your brain on drugs. Any questions?* I can't help it. There's basically nothing else to do but think about brains.

"So Anne," the doctor finally says, "do you have anything you'd like to ask me?" I don't. And I wouldn't know where to begin anyway. "Because there's no question you have Parkinson's Disease."

There's no question you have Parkinson's Disease.

I was hoping for better news. I know it's not his fault, but he may as well have murdered a unicorn right in front of me. A smasher of hope. And rainbows.

This is why I can't stand doctor visits. If you're at the doctor's, you can pretty much assume something's wrong. Sometimes I find myself rehearsing for the bad news I know is coming:

Thank you, Doctor, for the diagnosis. Is there a support group I can join? I'd like to get in touch with other people who are living and thriving with Parkinson's, so I can stay positive. I know modern medicine has made great strides. If Michael J. Fox can do it, so can I!

I wouldn't want to freak anyone out with the appropriate response, which would include furiously shaking my fist at the sky, shouting and cursing at whoever's up there screwing things up for me and then possibly throwing up. But it's not my style to emotionally fall apart, even though I've just been told, by a third doctor, that I have an awful, incurable neurological disease, at forty-five. And that's not the only thing he says.

"I'm prescribing a new medication for you. You're way too young to be going through this. Most patients I see in your condition are well over sixty." Awesome.

He goes on to tell me to stick with my yoga practice. I tell him it's been difficult. I do not mention that I've been making up excuses to get out of the end of class, like it's frog dissection day in tenth-grade science lab. One day I was expecting an important phone call. Another time I had to meet up with my husband somewhere. Once I just left without saying a word. Anything to escape the threat of being touched lightly on the face or the shoulders by the teacher coming around with essential oils. There's just no easy way to say "please don't touch me, and don't ask me why" without sounding like a snotty bitch.

Three years. That's how long this has been going on now. A thousand days in a row of what the fuck.

I leave the doctor's office with the new prescription and drive across the street to the car wash where I can sit and not think about how screwed I am. While I'm in there I briefly consider buying myself a "get well" card, or maybe a super tacky purse. I end up deciding on an Orange Gatorade.

From there I take the long way home, all the way down Ventura Boulevard from Encino to Toluca Lake in my convertible. It's beautiful outside, and I'm cruising along, hair flying in the wind, blaring The Stones. *Yeah, baby, that's me behind those Foster Grants*. If you saw me in that moment, you'd think I didn't have a care in the world.

Next stop: the pharmacy (another place I can't stand, in light of the fact that you're usually there because something's wrong). I hand them the new prescription. I then stand there staring at the at-home HIV testing kits, wondering what their accuracy percentage is and why would you take a chance either way.

Just then, Ike the pharmacist comes out from the pill-counting area and takes me aside.

"Do you know about the IV drip?" he asks me.

No, I don't know about the IV drip and believe me, in spite of all my tattoos, I really, really hate needles. But apparently people like me are getting "fantastic results with the IV drip" and here's a pamphlet.

"Look," he says. "We gotta take care of this thing. We can't have you walking around like this. You're way too young."

You know what? He's right. I *am* too young. Maybe it's time I start acting like it. I should go straight home, pour myself a big ol' bowl of Cap'n Crunch and paint my nails with Liquid Paper. This might be the perfect thing. I really don't dig responsibility of any kind, I don't always recycle, and sometimes I find myself wishing I could drop everything, jump in my car without packing and go find a commune in San Francisco where I can live. And when I do, you can all call me Rhiannon. That's my hippie name.

But here I am with what can easily be described as an uncool, unhip, lame-ass brain disease, possibly thanks to too much exposure to some or all of the following: processed sugar, processed food, booze, toxic chemicals, metals, stress, bad air, lead, fillings, chi flowing the wrong way, parasitic intestinal blockages and/or a glutathione deficiency. Google it, and you'll find a different answer every time. Once I found a website that said it was imperative I stop using toilet paper. That's the day I quit Googling stuff.

What I *have* learned, however (other than that the Internet is full of bad advice), is no matter what's going on, life is not meant to be a montage of catastrophes. It's also not a giant prison, and neither are these bizarre, meaty casings we are housed in for the time being. And they'd make terrible ones anyway. These bodies aren't exactly built to last. They get sick and get old and fall apart. But truth is, the me that is me is not the sick one here. And I refuse to feel imprisoned.

Maybe I'm not the perfect, stainless being I was when I came into the world. Maybe I've screwed up along the way and made some horrible decisions and maybe I still don't make sense to myself sometimes. And yeah, my brain's a little bit broken. But you will never hear me refer to myself as broken. And don't even get me started on the "what's wrong with me's." "What's wrong with me" is the hell spawn of self-deprecation and self-doubt. "What's wrong with me" is pointless and limiting. Whatever made this world and everything in it isn't wrong, it's miraculous. Typos are wrong. That's about it. And there's nothing wrong with you either.

We've all had our fair share of calamity and crap and hurt. We all know what it is to want to start over, to go back to the days of running around barefoot in the sprinklers waiting for your turn on the Slip 'N Slide. The easy days. The days in life before "the collapse." We've all felt a little incompetent, insufficient, overexposed, hopeless, unlovable, terrified, defective, unfit, and unsung at times. And deep down, for whatever reason, you might even think you deserve to. Because *why else would you be feeling that way.* Like the world is laughing at you.

I promise you it's not.

I remember the first time I met my friend Gretchen. There she stood by the front desk before my yoga class, a full five feet and ten inches of gorgeousness. I also remember how long it took her to fill out the form with her name and address, and then I found out why. Next to the question "Do you have any health issues?" she had written the longest list imaginable of diseases and problems to exist in one human body, and in the clearest penmanship I'd ever seen. Lupus. Ulcerative Colitis. Reynaud's Syndrome. Rheumatoid Arthritis. Scoliosis. Asthma. A cervical spinal fusion. Shoulder surgery.

Gretchen is happy. I've never known a person with that many things awry who laughed so easily. And it isn't because things for her aren't ableist and unfair and sucky, because they are. It's because sometimes, when the worst has happened, when you get the phone call with the bad news or the positive test results, you realize your feet are still on the ground. The dogs still need their dinner bowls, the laundry still needs to get done, and *Rocky* is still your favorite movie. It's because laughing about it all is so much more fun than crying in the corner. Screw. That.

To be in this world is a phenomenal thing. And sometimes that fact will hit you out of the blue when you least expect it, like when you're at the market, minding your own business, trying to decide what kind of coffee to get when you hear "Don't Stop Believin'" come on and you become suddenly, wholly consumed with everything that is beautiful about just being awake and being alive. I'm talking tears in your eyes and your heart broken wide open with love and amazement for it all, no matter what it looks like, when you realize the ultimate reality that lies not just within this life, but beyond it.

I finally make it home the day of the neurologist.

And you know how in the movies, someone will walk in the door with bad news and crumble in an inconsolable, sobbing heap? That's not what happens. My boxer dogs with their little zig-zagging bodies are right there to greet me, as always, and my husband is in the kitchen cooking dinner for us. I put the Stones on the stereo, a little "Sympathy for the Devil," and start dancing around the living room with the dogs while the broccoli is sizzling and my husband is asking, "What do you want to drink with dinner?"

And I'm filled with so much gratitude for my life, it's unreal.

The stories in this book are my experience. They're about life and yoga and illness and love and disaster and happiness. And since you're holding it, I'm hoping you relate in some way because A) that's the whole point, and B) we all need someone to relate to. And maybe a hand up (but with words). Because sometimes you just need to hear it's all going to work out, even though life may have whammed you and half the time everything might seem like a big fat mess and not at all what it's supposed to look like, which makes no sense in the first place since none of us *really* know what's going to happen and you can't change fate. If I could, I wouldn't have Parkinson's and

Prince would still be alive. These stories are for you.

Think about your life. Think about your own stories, about who you were a year ago, five years ago, half your lifetime ago. Chances are your mind will either go to something really beautiful, or something really painful. Maybe both. Or maybe you'll see a stranger, someone different who wears different clothes and has different answers. Don't judge them for it. They're learning. I'm learning. Look at all of us, learning. It's working out already.

Maybe you, too, live with an annoying disease. Or you have some kind of health concern you haven't had checked out yet because you fear the worst. Be afraid, but go anyway. You might be right. And maybe you do yoga, maybe not, maybe it means as much to you as *mamase-mamasa-mamakusa*. It's not like I hang out all day in Eka Pada Sirsasana with my left leg casually slung over my shoulder. I'm not hopping a bus to Kathmandu anytime soon. I've never even owned a passport. I'm an L.A. chick who grew up half a world away from India. I've met only one swami in my life, who actually quit being a swami because he was only twenty-two at the time and he decided he'd rather chase women (his words). I know I'm as West as it gets. But I'm here to tell you, yoga saved the ass of a girl who was once so high on mushrooms I lit my hair on fire by accident at a Depeche Mode concert. Then the Parkinson's thing started happening. Now I get up at 5:15 in the morning to teach 6:00 a.m. yoga classes.

Wanna come?

Nothing is so painful to the human mind
as a great and sudden change.

—MARY SHELLEY, *Frankenstein*

AFRAID

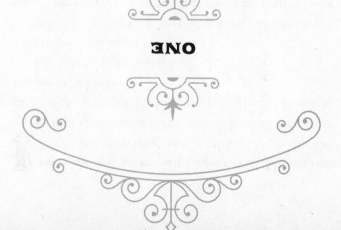

ONE

It was nothing at first. Just a little twitch. My left ring finger was twitching, slowly, almost languidly, the way a fishing line does when you've hooked something without any strength. Like a baby perch. I hadn't even gotten out of bed yet.

My first thought: stress?

(Nope, think again.)

It had to be. Working five nights a week in a bar really takes it out of you, especially when you're not getting home until three in the morning. And you can never go straight to sleep. First, you have to check your entire apartment for murderers. I never know what I'll do if I actually find one, but I do it anyway. Then I peel my grubby bar clothes off with my grenadine-spackled hands, throw some old sweats on and lie in bed watching repeats of *Law & Order: SVU*. Hopefully I fall asleep before the sun comes up.

This has been my life for six years. Or maybe seven. I've lost count.

I certainly don't feel any different, considering I've effectively woken up with an indication of brain damage. A little exhausted maybe, but there's nothing new about that. As far as I know everything's normal. I feel like anyone would feel, not knowing they've managed to cross an invisible line overnight, the one I sometimes imagine was the work of some rogue god, searing my life into two very distinct parts: Before The Horror/After The Horror. Maybe he was bored. Thanks, dude.

At the moment I'm just cozily lying in bed up in my huge and fantastic Hollywood Hills apartment, the one I insist on living in even though I can barely afford it. I sling drinks for a living. If you look in my refrigerator, you'll find nothing but leftover Thai food and maybe an old jar of horseradish. Around noonish I'll take my boxer Shamus McDog to the park up Beachwood Canyon and flirt with guys. I go to yoga three times a week, sometimes four. I enjoy horror movies, shopping for cheap shit on eBay and reading Charles Bukowski. I've been told I look like Jamie Lee Curtis and I talk like Courtney Love. I'm forty-two years old and I am a Scorpio.

And there isn't one single reason this morning to think my little life, as I know it, will never again be the same.

Except for the twitch.

Why sweat it, I decide. I'm not in the mood to get all riled up and start Googling stuff. That would entail way more effort than I'm willing to give it. Also, the same kind of thing happened once before right near my eye and it went away in, like, a day.

I'll just go to yoga. It'll be fine.

(Yeah, not exactly.)

This is the phase they call "early onset." I'm sure

there's a much scarier sounding Latin-based word for it but I have no idea what it is. I tend to zone out when I hear doctors say words I don't understand, mostly because they're talking about my broken brain and the whole thing gives me the creeps. They might as well be describing an autopsy.

But here's the great news: of all the shitty diseases out there, Parkinson's is definitely one of the slower moving ones. It's pretty much the slug of diseases, except maybe typhoid fever, and who gets that anymore. So I should probably be happy. At least it was kind enough to let me ease into the situation. But a warning would have been nice. *Live it up while you can, baby, because pretty soon something really bad is going down.*

And live it up I would. I'd live it up so big. Just think, I could have real coffee again! (Caffeine is a problem. It makes things ten times worse. Never hand me a Red Bull.) I'd go to the kitchen right this second and make myself the hugest, most caffeinated pot of coffee you've ever seen. Then I'd pour myself some in one of those ridiculously oversized cups that look like they're made for soup and saunter around my house with it. Or maybe I'd just stand there holding it like someone in an old Folgers' ad. *Mmmm... Smell that mountain grown aroma.* For some reason when I picture this, I'm also wearing a long, leopard-print silk robe and curlers in my hair. Apparently I'm a bored housewife from 1960 in this scenario. Which is fine with me. I'd give almost anything nowadays just to be a bored housewife.

So generally speaking, early onset means you start showing symptoms before the age of fifty. Some even say sixty. More likely seventy. Barely anyone gets it at forty-two, which puts me in approximately the top four percent of my class. *Winning.*

But no matter what your age, this is what it's like for pretty much everyone: weird shit starts happening for no apparent reason. You're not sick, you haven't visited any countries where you could have picked up a strange bacterial infection and you're probably not possessed by a demon. And something starts twitching. Usually it's a limb, but in some cases it's your head. Or your muscles might feel stiff. Or you start losing your balance. But you don't really care, mostly because it's easier not to, and because it's never happened before so it's not like this is a pattern here. As far as you know, your brain is working just fine.

Except it's not. And it hasn't been for quite some time. This is the day you know your dopamine-producing neurons have officially started to flat line. You are now operating on a scant twenty percent. And there's no getting it back.

Dopamine is a neurotransmitter that relays information between your neurons, information like memories
and images and thoughts. And it makes you feel good. This
is why things like exercise and heroin are so addicting,
because both produce dopamine. And when you don't have
enough, your neurons can't communicate like they should.
One will send a signal, which ends up floating in space and
not reaching the other one.

Knock, knock.

Who's there?

No one.

No one who?

Parkinson's Disease.

Later that day I come home from the dog park and collapse
on the couch. It's warm out. Gorgeous, actually. If Shamus
could talk, I'm sure he'd say it was the perfect ball-chasing
weather. (It always is.)

I love taking care of this uncomplicated little creature.
He's got soul. I could lie there all day and listen to the
sound of his pant.

Oh, and the twitch? Still there.

And now I'm thinking, watch. I have some kind of
horrible disease.

(Ding ding ding.)

I have never had health problems. I'm lucky. I've never even broken a bone. Once every five years or so I get strep throat and that's about it. I did step on a rusty nail one night at work, which jabbed itself right through my shoe and punctured my big toe, so it did occur to me I could have had lockjaw but in my finger. Or maybe it was just poor circulation. Bad air will cause all kinds of problems, and L.A. is really smoggy. It's a wonder everyone around here doesn't wake up twitching.

In a few hours I'll take a nap—if not I'll get cranky—and get ready for work in my finest *Coyote Ugly* outfit. Something will be hurriedly eaten on my way out the door that normally would not constitute dinner, like a muffin. Then I'll say goodbye to Shamus, who will hate me for leaving because he'll think I'm never coming back, even though I've explained to him many times *I have to go to work because someone has to pay the bills*, and zoom down to the bar by 8:00 p.m.

Two things will hit me when I walk in the door: the smell of floor cleanser, and the fact that I'm going to be stuck in this job for the rest of my life. I will try not to choke on either of them.

I don't want to be there. I'm sick of it and people are assholes. The other night some idiot actually chucked a beer bottle right by my head. But it's familiar, and I hate upheaval, and also I know of no other job where you're allowed to scream obscenities at people. Which is exactly what I did to the bottle guy. (He did apologize, saying, "I didn't see you." Fair enough.)

Here in L.A., everyone assumes if you're a bartender you must have moved here from somewhere else to be an actor. This is slightly annoying when you're actually *from* L.A., but once I gave it a shot. I can't say I got very far, but I did play a black jack dealer in a very terrible movie called *Angels of the City* directed by Freddie "Boom Boom" Washington from *Welcome Back Kotter*. The plot: *College girls dressed as hookers for a sorority initiation ceremony are kidnapped by pimps.* My scene was filmed in the middle of the night in a club in a crack neighborhood near downtown and I made $75. Nothing much happened with the acting thing after that. I had peaked.

But what I really want—what I've wanted for how long now?—is to teach yoga. I don't know what's stopping me. I'm already certified. I have two hundred hours of yoga training to my name, and the fancy piece of paper to prove it. It's the kind you frame with your name calligraphed in gold-flecked paint and a wax embossment. I'd hang it, but I put it somewhere for safekeeping and I have no clue where.

The one teaching interview I did go on was a slight disaster. I walked in, took one look at the other teachers waiting and totally Flashdanced myself. There I was with my no experience, feeling like a welder among real ballerinas in my khakis and my frizzy hair, all afraid I couldn't cut it. I probably should've hopped on my bicycle right then and ridden back to the steel plant, except really I'd be getting in my banged-up old Jetta and going back to the bar like the chickenshit I was. But I stayed. I stayed because GODDAMMIT, I'M GONNA BE A YOGA TEACHER AND I'M NOT GONNA BE AFRAID!

No, I did not get that teaching job.

Nor did I know at the time what fear really was.

Not even close.

But hey, who needs a "grown up" job with a regular paycheck and no beer bottles whizzing by your head. My life rules. I ran away with the circus. *I'm living the dream.*

The hour before the bar opens is always hectic, and no one is ever ready. Bands do their sound checks, ice gets delivered, liquor bottles get stocked. Invariably someone will lose something important and will stomp around yelling about it. Everyone tends to start off in various states of disgruntled.

And me? Don't worry about me. I'll be spending the next half hour cutting limes.

Afraid

This may sound sad, but this is my favorite part of my night. There's something very Zen about cutting limes. You can be having the worst day ever, but it won't matter when your entire focus is absorbed with slicing the perfect lime wedge. You're just *chop chop chopping*. And that's it. They should make people with anxiety do it. Then again, most people I know who work in bars do have anxiety. I wonder why.

Kierkegaard said, "If you look at things very closely, you'll forget that you're going to die." I'd say that about sums it up. I'm just going to stand there and turn four pounds of round green fruit into garnish for hipsters to squeeze into their gin and tonics. It will be a remarkable display of my potential as a human being.

I grab the first of the limes and set it on the cutting board. And right when I go to stab its skin, something distracts me.

The twitch.

Fuck.

And so it began. Let the record show Friday, April 3, 2009, deserves nothing less than a big black Sharpie'd X on it with a skull on top, denoting the imminent demise of Anne Clendening's dopamine. Lock the doors and close all the windows, honey. Things are about to get funky.

Weeks go by. It gets worse. And by worse I mean what started as a finger twitch can easily now be described as a bit more of a hand flutter, which is slightly less ignorable but I manage to do it anyway. That way it doesn't exist.

Am I concerned? Not really. I'm way too busy ignoring it.

Now I'm a sixteen-year-old girl who somehow manages to remain in denial of her recent weight gain until a baby ends up falling out of her in the middle of prom.

No, I do not discuss it with anyone. Not friends, not family. No one. There's nothing to discuss, as you can tell by my Facebook posts which remain super casual and not at all indicative of a crisis.

"Did anyone just feel that earthquake?"

"Who wants to meet me at yoga?"

"Sitting at home, listening to *Dark Side of the Moon...*"

Fortunately—if you can say that—the problem is in my left hand, which is the hand I'm completely inept with anyway. So at this point, my plan is to keep on ignoring it. Forever. And since it doesn't seem particularly life-threatening, I figure there's no need to go spend money I don't have with some quack who'll charge me up the ass to lecture me about the evils of stress and send me away with an informative handout. Again, I already know it's stress, which is exactly what I said the first twenty times someone noticed. Either that, or I'd had too much coffee. Once I told someone I'd just banged my hand in the car door. Usually I'll say it's nothing and strut away. Because *nothing can crack this bitch*.

One night I go to yoga for the first time since this mysterious thing inside me saw fit to show up and wreck everything. I needed to feel a sense of normalcy again, since normal is the first thing to fly out the window when your hand starts moving all on its own, and *normally* I'd be there anyway, and even though things were definitely not what anyone would call "normal," I make myself go.

I stomp into class and throw my mat down with a thunk. This says, *I command you, yoga, to make this go away*. I don't care where. It's just got to go. It's the lingering houseguest you never invited over in the first place. Persona non grata.

Class starts. And somewhere between the opening meditation and the time we're in Down Dog, which couldn't have been more than twelve minutes later, I notice it. The fluttering has stopped. It's actually *stopped*. And what's even more of a miracle is that I'm not even questioning it. I'm just there, moving and breathing and wringing all the unease from the past few weeks out of my malfunctioning body, all happy, totally in the moment, wishing I could glue it down and toss around in it forever.

Was it a fluke? Probably not. And it doesn't matter. I'm just glad it happened.

One night I'm behind the bar. And it's slammin' in there. It's all music and people and money. A very hot, Abercrombie and Fitch–looking dude walks up to the bar and asks me for a Kamikaze, the easiest drink in the world to make. And I cannot think of what goes in it. Vodka, that's all I know. Or is it lemon vodka? And wait, what else? (*Finger snap. Finger snap.*) No idea.

"Hey Kelly," I say to the other bartender, "What's in a Kamikaze again?"

And Kelly looks at me like, "Really?"

Yes, really.

And now I'm getting scared.

I'm getting scared because this isn't the first time this has happened.

I'm getting scared because this is starting to get ridiculous.

I'm getting scared because my parents had about a million health problems between them and now it's my turn.

Afraid

I'm getting scared because no one will want to spend the rest of their life with me if this gets any worse.

I'm getting scared because my body is failing at being a body.

I saw *The Exorcist* when I was twelve. I do not scare easily.

Oh, and one more thing: I hate it for making me scared.

Fear is a bastard. Fear is an attention whore. I want to ask fear if it has mommy issues, because that's the only reason I can think why it needs attention so bad. I want fear to get Parkinson's. Then maybe fear will know how it feels to be on the run from something it doesn't understand.

The worst part of any problem, especially health problems, is the fear of the unknown. I can't tell you how many times I've woken up in a cold sweat thinking I'm being chased by a grunting, disfigured man wielding a hatchet. Usually we're at an abandoned campground, which leads me to believe this is a subconscious mashup of *Friday the 13th* and *The Texas Chainsaw Massacre*. He never catches me. The only thing that ever happens is I'm running and he's chasing. It's pretty horrible. I know it's not real, but it feels real, and you know how feelings are. They make everything real.

But I will carry on like nothing's up. I will do everything a human can possibly do to shun this grim reality of my ever-worsening condition in hopes it will magically disappear.

Some people—bless their sweet hearts and all—will tell me I'm "sticking my head in the sand," that something is obviously wrong and maybe I should go to the doctor. And I will swiftly shut them up by telling them they worry too much.

Besides. It was bound to stop.

Right?

(Wrong.)

There is no way this is happening.

Scientists and people on acid claim reality is an illusion and they'd better be right. Because this was some bullshit. It wasn't even a regular problem. Maybe if it were something else more common, like a mole that had suddenly turned black, I wouldn't be feeling like such an oddity. But I'd never met anyone whose hand started fluttering out of the blue.

Two months after it all started I secretly decide to go see the doctor. If no one knows, then no one can ask me how it went, because now I have a brain tumor. This suddenly became clear when I made the appointment. I imagine the doctor will want to do some kind of super invasive exam, after which he'll confirm the presence of an inoperable mass that's causing the problem, and that I should really think about telling my loved ones "sooner rather than later" that I am indeed dying. Hopefully I'll have enough time to get my affairs in order.

The lobby of Dr. Schnaufer's office is one of those lobbies that tries to appear cheerful but fails. The walls are beige, the trim is mauve and the Cézanne-inspired paintings on them are pointless. The last time I was there I had the flu, maybe a year earlier. And the time before that, I don't remember. Maybe that was it. I'm healthy and I'd really like to stay that way, thanks.

I check in, have a seat, and wait for my doom.

"Anne?"

Okay, that was awfully fast.

The nurse leads me into the exam room. Two minutes later Dr. Schnaufer comes in, who looks exactly like Woody Allen with a stethoscope. I wonder if people tell him that.

"So Anne, what brings you in?"

I tell him about the hand thing, which he looks at.

"And how long has it been happening?"

"Two months," I say, hoping I don't get scolded for waiting so long. I search his face for a look that might say, *Oh it's nothing.* Or, *you're fucked.* But there is no look one way or the other. They must go through special training.

Then comes the next question, which I was not prepared for. "Tell me, do you have a history of drug or alcohol abuse?"

Do I have a history of drug or alcohol abuse? That's the second thing he asks? *How dare you, sir!*

"What would that have to do with it?"

"Well, it causes brain damage, for one thing. Especially if you were young."

My eyes turn into a squint. I'm half tempted to rattle off the Pythagorean theorem to prove him wrong. But it's possible he wasn't.

When you start thinking about what your life was like ten years ago—and not in general terms, but in highly specific detail—it's disturbing to realize how certain elements of your being are completely dead. They die long before you do. It's astonishing to consider all the things from your past that used to happen all the time but (a) never happen anymore, and (b) never even cross your mind. It's almost like those things didn't happen. Or maybe it seems like they just happened to someone else. To someone you don't really know. To someone you just hung out with for one night, and now you can't even remember her name.

—CHUCK KLOSTERMAN

TWO

TROUBLED

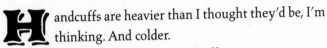andcuffs are heavier than I thought they'd be, I'm thinking. And colder.

And: Is this really necessary? Cuffs?

Also: God that guy is hot.

The hot guy and I are handcuffed to the same bench at the West L.A. Police Station. He's talking to the police, something about a bar fight. I'd been in a spontaneous drag race on Sunset Boulevard with some other hot guy in a BMW. I think it was a BMW. It was definitely white. That's about all I can tell you.

There's something about it, the sight of a bloody and battered man in restraints. I dug it. What a hottie. He probably had a hot name, too, like Bowie. And what if Bowie and me hooked up? We'd have the cutest story ever, that's what!

How'd we meet, you ask? Well, I was twenty-one years old, and I'd just gotten nailed for drunk driving with three existing bench warrants for my arrest. And when they hauled me in, Bowie was sitting there, looking all cute in his torn Izod shirt, and when we locked eyes we both just knew.... Now we live together right on the beach. Bowie surfs all day while I work on my tan and sip on little pink drinks like Malibu Barbie.

Before I can shamelessly throw myself at hot bar-fight-guy, they take him away, I assume to get booked.

It's like a screwed up form of speed dating. Dammit, there went my new fella.

Now what. How long have I been there? An hour already? Someone is screaming. Who would be screaming in a police station? Oh I see, it's a prostitute. A prostitute is screaming. This may be my first time, but I know that can't possibly be acceptable. I watch *21 Jump Street*. Not a lot of screaming in *21 Jump Street*.

I don't belong there. I don't belong in jail with prostitutes. Prostitutes are rough and trampy, and I'm from West L.A. This is nothing but a waste of everyone's time, and if anyone has a shred of decency they'd take these damn cuffs off already because they're really starting to get on my nerves.

"Excuse me," I ask the air, "can someone please take these handcuffs off?"

Nothing.

God. I asked nicely.

Well then. Might as well get comfy, I think. Taking off my shoes seems like a good start. Although it takes some doing when you don't have the use of your hands and all. Somehow I manage to wiggle one of my Doc Martens halfway off with the toe of the other by the time a policeman comes walking up.

Finally, someone to talk to! I have the perfect opening

line. "Hey, are there, like, any bullets in that gun ya got there?"

I sound like a saloon girl. I slur with Long Islands.

He keeps walking. How very smug.

I get it. This is the part where I'm supposed to sit there and think about what I've done. Maybe reevaluate my "life choices." Drum up some remorse. Well, everyone is sadly, sadly mistaken if they think I'm about to quit drinking. I don't want to hear it, not even a whiff. They could suggest it all they wanted, but suggesting I quit drinking would be like suggesting I shave my head. Or I peel my own skin off. Because that's how obscenely wrong and out of the fucking question it is at this point.

Three a.m. rolls around by the time my angry and disappointed parents finally pick me up from the slammer. It's bad. And not the yelling kind of bad—the *silent* kind. Bad silence is the worst. When you render your own parents speechless with your behavior, that's how you know you've really fucked up, and two quietly seething parents are no match for me in such a state. That being: drunk.

The torture lasts halfway home. Finally, my mother, with zero regard for my feelings, has exactly one thing to say. "You should have seen yourself, all drunk, flirting with the cops."

What a masterful belittling. I had to hand it to her. I think I may have even clapped.

Lesson learned: next time, take the side streets home.

I wasn't exactly in a rush to find yoga at twenty-one years old. When you're in the clutches of a drinking problem you don't really sit around thinking, *I should really knock this shit off and go get my Eastern philosophy on.* On your to-do list, pursuing a higher state of consciousness doesn't really rank. It's more like, *put on* Led Zeppelin 4 *and pass me some of that Root Beer Schnapps.*

This was the eighties. The "New Age" decade. People were wearing crystals and patchouli oil and swearing by Transcendental Meditation. The whole thing put a bad taste in my mouth. I thought it was for the weak-minded, the lonely, the friendless. The *desperate.* Oh, and Shirley MacLaine. Maybe you remember the book *Out on a Limb?* The one she wrote about her encounters with trance channelers and extraterrestrials? I rest my case.

But hey, if you and your cult buddies felt the need to get together and cling to your pseudo-philosophies, I certainly wasn't going to stop you. You could burn your incense and grow your dreadlocks all you wanted. Or better yet, maybe you could grab your tambourine and go whoop it up with the Hare Krishnas who sang and danced at the airport! Because that's what the world needed. *More hippies.*

You never see that anymore. Maybe people complained. I never knew if it was some kind of recruitment technique or they were just having fun, but you had to assume they were either brainwashed or on psychotropic drugs. Most likely both. This was clearly a bad combo and something to be avoided because, as my brother used to tell me, *that's how Charles Manson got girls like me to be into his family.* I didn't want to end up with a murder rap and an X carved into my forehead.

(Obvious side note: I changed my mind about yoga. Ten years later, to be exact. I even own a tambourine.)

Drinking, however, was a different story. Or two, depending how you look at it. I once saw Carrie Fisher describe what she *thought* drinking would be like, having grown up in the sixties with show business parents who, by the sound of it, may actually have raised her within the confines of a piano bar. And the way she described it, she held out her hand like she was holding a martini glass, threw her head back and let out a very loud and lengthy cackle as if to say, "Dahling! Isn't life just *smashing*!"

She was, of course, wrong. And so was I.

I wanted to be a writer, and writers drank. They sat at

their typewriters in their Laurel Canyon bungalows with their whiskey and their overflowing ashtrays and got to hang out with the likes of Timothy Leary and Fleetwood Mac because *that's how interesting they were*. My lack of self-restraint would be perceived as charming, a sure sign of my writing talent. All my friends would be cool. I'd get invited to dinners at Spago and all the best funerals. Maybe Andy Warhol would paint me.

Exactly two of those things happened: the writing and the drinking. Except it was bad writing and too much drinking. Or maybe too much writing and bad drinking. Either way, in the words of Caroline Knapp from her amazing-in-a-brutal-way memoir *Drinking: A Love Story*, it was a "slow, gradual, insidious, elusive *becoming*." And it ended up nothing like the way it started.

I'm fourteen years old, standing in our very seventies light blue kitchen, eyeing the emerald green bottle of Cutty Sark up in the liquor cabinet. There are details to memorize: The placement of the bottle on the shelf, which direction the ship on the label is facing, the whole scene.

No one's home. Go for it.

I take it down and hold it awkwardly, the way you might hold a deceptively heavy trophy. I put a crystal glass on the counter that seems vaguely appropriate, the one with the three initials etched into it: WEC, my father. The sounds are exhilarating. The spinning of the cap uncapping, the chime of the bottle when it touches the crystal. Dreamy, even. Like rainfall. All the while I'm listening for the dreaded crack of the front door. When you're fourteen, the last thing you want is for anyone to barge in on you while you're helping yourself to the Scotch.

I pour a little in the glass, just enough, and cut it with a little Mountain Dew. Then I dribble a little water into the bottle and oh so carefully place it back in the cabinet exactly the way I found it.

I know what I'm doing. It's not my first time.

Cocktail in hand, I go out to the backyard and sneak behind the bushes, like a spy. I'm James Bond in tube socks and Dolphin shorts. Then I drink the firewater.

It baffled me knowing some people didn't like the taste of alcohol. There must have been something wrong with their tongues. They didn't know what they were missing. One sip, and bam. I was a god. Invincible. And it tasted good. Top that.

No, I'm not getting beaten at home. Nobody ever locked me in an attic and no weirdo ever touched me. I'm not being neglected. Honestly, I'm not even sure where I got the idea. My parents barely drank. That bottle of Cutty

Sark was, in fact, a little dusty.

The Clendenings were married in 1959 and that's where they stayed. He was a lawyer, and the dad you want: Honest. Sharp-witted. Sentimental. Think Gregory Peck in *To Kill a Mockingbird*, except without the Southern accent. Or Gregory Peck period. They had a boy, John, my brother. Little Annie made four. And my Mia Farrow-looking mother with her slight frame and her pixie haircut stayed home and took care of us all.

Dinner is served! She'd announce every night at 7:00, when a tuna casserole would be presented. This would be done with pride.

The kitchen is closed, she'd announce an hour later, in time to watch *Ironside.*

Sound normal? It was. Unbelievably so. If you lifted me out of my life and dropped me into an episode of *Happy Days*, I probably wouldn't have noticed.

Tonight, on a Very Special Episode:
Anne Gets into the Cutty Sark and Guzzles It in the Bushes.

One minute, I'm a tragically average, fair and freckled eighth grader with algebra homework. The next, I'm one who has swallowed liquor. I'm a rebel. *I'm a line crosser.*

Do I worry about where it'll take me? Please. It's just harmless fun, not *Go Ask Alice*. Besides, I'm too busy rebelling. What I'm rebelling against, I have no idea. Parents, rules, take your pick. Fuck if I knew. *Now watch me flip my Farrah hair as I crack open a can of Pabst Blue Ribbon with my tongue.*

It takes balance. You learn to straddle worlds. *Good Girl/Lush.* Just act accordingly, and whatever you do don't mix them up. You definitely don't want to show up to family dinners wearing heavy black eyeliner and a ripped Siouxsie and the Banshees T-shirt. Save that look for later, when you split early and head over to the Sunset Strip with your friend Katie Scott. And don't forget the Aqua Net. That hair isn't going to stay crimped all on its own. (Again. The eighties.)

Sometimes I wonder if I could have "stopped in time," seeing how I wasn't quite developing very many "necessary life skills," much less "living up to my potential" according to the comments on every report card I ever got. But when you're that young, you don't really care. Or at least I didn't. Maybe I would have if the future me had the capability to appear in a hologram to warn the young me that if I kept this up, things would eventually go south and that one day I'd be sitting in a doctor's office being told I may have given myself permanent brain damage.

Young me wouldn't believe it anyway. I probably would have thrown a drink in my own face.

"I'll take a bottle of Peach Schnapps." I'm casual. I'm confident. I'm sixteen.

"Will that be all?"

Oh, hell no.

"...And a bottle of Smirnoff."

The liquor store in Koreatown sold to anyone. Even sixteen-year-olds with no ID in their Catholic school uniform. Apparently the guy behind the counter didn't recognize the blue plaid of Jesus when he saw it. Sucker. Totally worth the drive all the way across town.

It's amazing how fearless you can be when you want something bad enough, the lengths to which you'll go, the grit you'll put into the scheming and maneuvering. That's determination for you. I would have made a good bounty hunter.

As long as I didn't get caught, that is. *Must not get caught.*

"Anne, we have to talk to you."

There they were, my parents, standing at the foot of my bed one morning, their arms crossed and their bodies stiff, like the two lost members of Run-DMC. They were on to me. I'd come home from a house party in Hancock Park the night before, thrown up, and passed out for who knows how long on the bathroom floor. Seventeen years old now, and I've started to get sloppy. At least that floor was carpeted.

My mother did the talking. "Anne, about the drinking."

Uh oh. Here we go.

"It's out of control. You went to the beach the other day and came home at four o'clock smelling of alcohol! And last night? WHY IN GOD'S NAME ARE YOU BEHAVING LIKE THIS??!"

Never ask a person in the throes of a budding substance-abuse problem "why" anything. You'll get lied to, yelled at, maybe even kicked in the crotch. But these were my parents, and I had to be smart. So I deflect their questions the best way I know how, by making them doubt their own judgment.

"I think you're making a big deal out of nothing."

"And WE think you need to get your act together."

Whatever. I responded by slamming my bedroom door and blaring Black Sabbath. Because that'll show 'em.

That's me. Daughter of the year.

At least I wasn't in Katie Scott's shoes. Katie Scott got hauled off to rehab at St. John's after a particularly bad drinking binge with her boyfriend Daniel. Daniel was a "bad influence" who had been warned to stay away from Katie, but shortly after that, they were spotted together in Westwood tooling around on her moped and she got "sent away."

Consequences were now starting to happen to people. And it was making me very nervous.

Back in the eighties, rehab was cloaked in mystery. There were no depressing shows about interventions, no celebrity drug addicts. There was only a young Linda Blair in the TV movie of the week *Sarah T: Portrait of a Teenage Alcoholic*, a movie that only proved I *wasn't* an alcoholic because I didn't drink at school. I did see an interview with Elizabeth Taylor after she went to the Betty Ford Clinic and the whole thing sounded awful. Just like AA. There was another cult. What else would you call people huddled up in dimly lit church basements, jammering on about their problems in the name of *not drinking*? It had to be torture. I wasn't *that* bad. Maybe you were. Off you go!

A small and stupid part of me almost wished I had a reason for it. Nothing horrible, just something, anything I could point to and say, *This is why I'm doing this. It makes total sense.* But there wasn't so much as a sharp edge in sight to slam myself against and watch any logic spill out, like a piñata. There wasn't one thing I could point to, no definitive event that might explain it all. And that was the insidiousness of it. There was no *why*, and you can really drive yourself crazy with *whys*. I was already going slightly crazy, and it felt small, because it was, and the smallness was not only starting to get old, it was unoriginal. At least I was good at it.

Fuck it. I drain the Scotch.

Since it's impossible to fit the next five years into one chapter, I'll boil it down to this: a series of bad decisions coupled with utter confusion about my place in the world and what I was doing because I had a pretty strong hunch there was more to life than just avoiding rehab.

Addiction, at its worst, is akin to having Stockholm Syndrome. You're like a hostage who has developed an irrational affection for your captor. They can abuse you, torture you, even threaten to kill you, and you'll remain inexplicably and disturbingly loyal. *No worries. I'll just carry on.*

I had a checklist: I didn't hang out in alleys with bottles of Boone's Farm wrapped in brown paper bags. I never once woke up on a park bench under a pile of newspapers. My liver seemed to be in fine working order. It helps to picture the worst, most skid-row version of an alcoholic you can possibly think of so you can say, with all the certainty in the world, I AM NOT THAT AND I NEVER WILL BE.

Until something happens. Like you get arrested. And then still not realize how totally wrong you can be about your own fucking life.

One day you might walk into a bar in Venice called the Townhouse, plunk down a jarful of pennies, and ask for a pint of beer. Oh, and you're also barefoot. When the duly appalled bartender says pennies are unacceptable, you'll reason, "Dude, IT'S AMERICAN CURRENCY." You'll almost feel bad for putting him on the spot. Almost. You might even go so far as to offer to let him keep the jar. Again he'll say no, so you'll have no choice but to skulk out of there and find a liquor store up the street that'll take it. Then you'll show up for your father in the hospital barefoot *and* drunk right after he gets a tumor removed from his kidney and act like nothing's up, which is a challenge with all the bright and confrontational lighting.

Daughter of the decade.

The morning I wake up wearing my father's pajamas I know something incredibly bad must have gone down the night before, and I am of course right. Apparently my parents had to dress me when I got home. I remember none of it.

Where was I again?

Malibu. A restaurant in Malibu.

I peel myself away from the bed. It's noon-ish. In a daring move, and with every hope of staying inconspicuous—or at best, invisible—I slink down to the kitchen. No luck. There's my mother. And she's pissed.

"Anne…"

Busted. It's like *Midnight Express*.

"…you're going to St. John's."

Rehab? No way. I'd rather go to a Turkish prison.

"It's all arranged."

In other words, *you can do this the easy way or the hard way. Anne.* Clearly she had read some Al-Anon literature that said the best way to get an alcoholic to help themselves is to threaten them in a hungover moment of weakness the minute they wake up.

"Hold on." Panic. "I'll quit drinking. I'll go to meetings." Panic and ramble. This, coupled with the look, the one meant to be interpreted as *come on, you don't really want to drop me off at the hospital with the junkies and the crazies, do you?*

She buys it. I guess she missed the part where you're not supposed to make deals with said alcoholic.

"You have one chance. And that's it."

And something inside me says, *ya might wanna do this.*

The details are fuzzy, but I can tell you I sat in a meeting that night somewhere in the valley with my friend Sammy, feeling a combination of things I haven't had to feel since: Hungover. Defeated. And also a little drunk still.

"It's gonna be okay, Annie." Was it? Because it felt like ass. And what does that even mean, It's gonna be okay? It's like the welcome mat they put out for you when you arrive at the bottom. Broke? Suicidal? Did the cancer spread? *Hey, it's gonna be okay.* But he was right.

1989: the year I got sober.

And it all became the past.

There is a Zen saying, that life will give you what you need to awaken. And I think it's safe to say it's usually something painful and something that you don't want. Like an addiction. But here's the easy part of not drinking: not drinking. It's pretty simple, even though after all these years it does still occur to me every once in a while. *I know what I should do today. I should just get drunk.* Like an amputee might be compelled to scratch a phantom limb. (I imagine.) But liquor isn't really even the problem. The Jack Daniel's certainly isn't going to throw itself down your throat. It's just sitting there. I did take a sip of tequila not long ago thinking it was Red Bull. Surprise! It was Patron! *Oops.*

And the hard part? Not knowing who you are anymore. Because an addict newly separated from their thing, whether it's drinking, drugs, throwing up ten times a day, or anything else is like a person with no head. Your entire identity goes M.I.A. once you're no longer doing it. That's who you were, because that's what you did. Then you're just screwed, because it hurts to live with it just as much as it hurts to live without it, even though it's obvious that you should live without it because it's made your life hell. Or maybe you made your own hell. You're so confused at that point you have no idea what to think, and you're not always up for finding out. I'd much rather spend all day on the Santa Monica Pier playing Asteroids than delve into the murk and analyze myself. And if you think I haven't gone down to the pier to do that recently, well, you'd be wrong. Sometimes you just have to be twelve again.

Carl Jung, badass psychoanalyst, said that *there is no coming to consciousness without pain, that people will do anything, no matter how absurd, to avoid facing their own soul.* Maybe that's who we all are, in one way or another. A bunch of soul avoiders. And the things we do are totally absurd. But if I hadn't gone through all that, and if I hadn't gotten sober and stayed sober, I don't know if I ever would have shown up to my first yoga class, or if it would have even meant anything. All that matters anyway is what *did* happen. There is no "what if." "What if" is nothing but a bridge to nowhere. And I wouldn't change a thing.

Now if this were a made-up movie version of events, the story could have easily ended in that meeting. You'd see whoever was playing me sitting there smiling, and it would be a shy but hopeful smile, one that says, *You know, maybe it will be okay....* Then the camera would pan out to show all the people—the ones who aren't outside smoking—and a narrator would take it from there, possibly Morgan Freeman, summing it all up with something like this:

Anne never did go to rehab. It's been twenty-eight years since she sat in that meeting, and she hasn't had a drink since. (Which is true.) *And that was the end of her struggles.* (Which is not.)

He had two lives: one, open, seen and known by all who cared to know, full of relative truth and of relative falsehood, exactly like the lives of his friends and acquaintances; and another life running its course in secret. And through some strange, perhaps accidental, conjunction of circumstances, everything that was essential, of interest and of value to him, everything in which he was sincere and did not deceive himself, everything that made the kernel of his life, was hidden from other people.

—ANTON CHEKHOV,

The Lady with the Little Dog and Other Stories

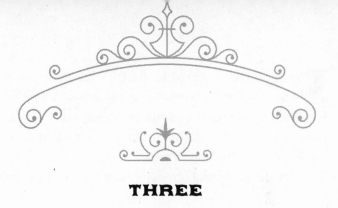

THREE

HIDDEN

I'm in exam room #2 waiting for Dr. Schnaufer to come back. It is not the most thrilling place on Earth. I've literally spent the last five minutes staring at a clear acrylic jar filled with cotton balls trying to guess how many are in there. (120, I'm thinking.) That's how bored I am.

"Stay here," he said fifteen minutes ago. "I'll be right back."

I have no idea where he went. I also don't think he cared enough about the tremor, which could either mean one of two things. Either he went to quietly call Cedars-Sinai to have me airlifted out of there and immediately rushed into surgery, or he knows it's nothing and he's preparing himself with a lecture about my lifestyle and what stress does to the body. And I will tell him I'll cool it on the processed sugar. Then he'll recommend a multi-vitamin, which I may or may not get, and I'll thank him for the advice. And that'll be that.

Just then the door opens. Dr. Schnaufer sashays back in, waving a printout. "Okay Anne!" he says. "It looks like you have something called essential tremor."

Wait, that's what he's been doing? *Googling it?*

"And what is essential tremor?"

It turns out essential tremor is a relatively common and manageable neurological condition that causes things like your hand or your head to shake and that's what

Katherine Hepburn had. (Although I'm not quite sure why they call it "essential." No one *needs* a tremor.) They don't know why some people get it. And right now I don't care.

"So it's no big deal."

"I wouldn't worry about it," he says. I always did like that Dr. Schnaufer. "But if you like, I can prescribe a medication that'll help."

Meds? No. Meds are the last thing I'd like.

Sick people take meds.

"Nope, I'll be fine, thanks."

And with that, I hop off the exam table and become the emoji for wind. In my mind I'm already back at home with Shamus and my nonthreatening, nontumor diagnosis. I am an echo.

I'll be fine…

    fine…

      fine…

"Oh, and Anne?" God. What now. "It couldn't hurt to get a second opinion. From a neurologist."

Dun dun duh.

Second opinion. Neurologist. There's three words you never want to hear together.

"Do I have to?"

"It's a good idea."

No it isn't. It's a terrible idea. They certainly don't

send you to the neurologist to get a second opinion for no reason. I'd never heard of anyone going to the brain doctor for "preventative measures." Cancer, yes. Aneurysms, yes. Beyond that I'm not sure.

He sends me off with the feeble printout and a referral. I don't want either. I feel like a dog who just got slapped on the nose for getting too excited.

I shuffle to the elevator and plunge to the ground level. There's been a shift. I'm a different person than I was when I got there an hour ago. An hour ago I wasn't a person who needed to see a neurologist, and now I *am* a person who needs to see a neurologist. And as I'm walking down the street I'm looking at others who probably *don't* need to see a neurologist, and envying them. They get to just hang out on Robertson Boulevard and have lunch. Or shop. They're probably shopping for Mercedes Benzes and antique light fixtures and baby strollers, which around here they call "prams." Because it's fancy.

And then I realize where I am. I'm right in front of a restaurant where I worked fifteen years earlier, only it's not that restaurant. It looks nothing like it used to. Before, it was beautiful and invitingly rustic. Now they've gone and changed it into a totally different restaurant that looks exactly like a bank.

A sign on the door reads, "For Lease." It is abandoned.

And now I want to cry.

Advice: when feeling down, be sure to not accidentally walk by a place from your young and relatively carefree past that doesn't look the same. And whatever you do, don't stand there with your sad eyes and your questionable hand tremor staring at the empty, subpar replacement thing getting all wrapped up in a tale of woe about how bitchin' your life was back in the day. It'll rip your heart right out. And hand you back an existential crisis.

I was twenty-seven then, four and a half years sober and bulletproof. Something like this was *never* going to happen to me. Not in a million lifetimes. Yet it was happening, much to my disbelief, which meant this very well *could be* my millionth lifetime, which is an incredibly humbling thought, and what are lifetimes anyway because twenty-seven was a decade and a half ago now and that alone feels like a lifetime, and where did everything go wrong.

I didn't need a neurologist. I needed a time machine. I needed to run around the past and gather up all the old, unbroken parts of me and try to Frankenstein myself back together again. My healthy body, my unjaded sixteen-year-old heart, my baby brain. I may not make such a pretty monster, but at least I'd feel like me again, which is pretty difficult when there's an evil force inside your body you have little to no control over. Sometimes I imagine this must be what it feels like to swallow lightning.

I believe in yoga this moment is called "completely missing the point of who you really are." Because even though they didn't have microscopes or much understanding of human anatomy four thousand years ago when the Yoga Sutras (the entire philosophy yoga is based on) were written, they're pretty clear: false identification happens when we mistake the mind and the body for the Self. Capital S. Because if that were the case, we'd be in big trouble. Something like three-quarters of the cells in your body get replaced every two and a half weeks and become dust. Millions of them just died in the last two seconds alone. And I don't know how they know all this, or how cells even have the intelligence to become an elbow or a stomach or whatever or how your skin lasts less than a month, but most of your body is not the same as it was five years ago. Or even five weeks ago. Yet, you're still you. You, the interminable being right smack in the middle of it all.

I didn't know who I was that day. I was in a hover, a person in between two other people, both me, both not me. Both felt far away. Both felt oddly close. I was interconnected to not much and not sure what to do about it, except to say go home and try not to flip out.

By the time I walk in the door I'm exhausted and it's only two o'clock. I immediately stash the printout (the one with the misdiagnosis) in a shelf between a bunch of books. You definitely don't want evidence of a morning like this casually lying around. Someone might come over and see it, and then what do you say. *Oh, that's just some info on my scary tremor.*

I then find it completely appropriate to pull the shades down, crawl into bed, and watch a marathon of *The Hills*.

Denial? Maybe a little.

And fuck it.

"You know, Brooke Shields sure hasn't aged very well."

It's a month later. My mother and I are on my couch watching Michael Jackson's funeral.

"Why do you say that?"

"You can tell by her neck. You can always tell by a woman's neck. Look at Susan Lucci."

I haven't told her yet about the doctor. Or the tremor. There's no need. I'm doing much better now that I know it's definitely nothing.

Which is what I chose to hear.

And why would you worry your own mother over nothing.

Besides, it's true. Oddly enough, it hasn't been bothering me as much. In fact, I actually feel kind of great. I'm the last person who needs to see a neurologist.

Sick people go to the neurologist.

Meanwhile, the printout is looming up on the shelf, like a killer lying in wait. I don't know why I didn't just throw it away. All I can hope is my mother doesn't get a sudden urge to read, which looks unlikely.

"Seriously. Brooke Shields looks like she's fifty."

Later, after talking my mother out of going downtown to crash Michael Jackson's funeral, I go to work. And it's great.

Everything is great.

Swear to god.

One night I'm in yoga. We're flowing. We're sweating. I'm not even thinking about the tremor.

Correction: I'm *trying* not to think about the tremor.

The feeling good thing didn't last very long.

Parkinson's is like your annoying neighbors who yell at each other and play music way too loud. You might tolerate it for a bit, until one day you get finally get sick of it and stomp over there and ask them to please stop it. And maybe things will quiet down for a day or two, and you'll think, *All right, glad they listened.* Then pretty soon the neighbors will start right back up again with the noise. Because they didn't listen. They were just out of town.

So I'm in yoga. Because fuck that tremor.

(The one I'm not thinking about.)

We're in Warrior One. We're facing the front of the room, one foot forward, knee bent, sword held high in the air. Warrior One is the embodiment of courage.

"Now imagine this," the teacher says. "Imagine something in front of you, something in your life that's a problem."

Gee. Let me think.

"Maybe it's a fear. Or maybe it's something about yourself you don't like. Or can't accept."

No prompting needed. But thanks.

"Now I want you to see it. Really see it...."

Oh, no worries, I see it. I really see it. And what I see is a hideous, throbbing blob of darkness. It is a mess. It is a malignancy.

"And on the count of three, I want you to take that sword, bring it down and cut that thing *right down the middle.*"

That's all she had to say. It was like a battle cry. In that moment, you couldn't tell me I didn't have an instrument of torture in my hands.

"One…"

I take an inhale.

"Two…"

My lungs fill with breath. I'm ready.

THREE!"

And the sword comes down.

Swoosh!

"Again!"

Swoosh!

"AGAIN!"

SWOOSH!

I wish I could tell you what it was like to see that thing collapse to the floor once I sliced it to ribbons. But you can't see anything when you're crying that hard.

One of the hardest things to do is give yourself permission to be in pain of any kind. There's a reason we have survival instincts, so that we *don't die.* That goes for humans, animals (redundant, I know), all the fishes in the sea, everyone. It's kind of universal. Some researchers say that even plants feel pain and that a cucumber will scream when you cut it. (And some others say that's crap because they have no brain or central nervous system.) The point is, we're all wusses. And emotional pain is the worst. Avoid it too long, and it'll shove its way right in, which ends up way more painful than if you just went ahead and felt that pain to begin with. But you don't get to be called a warrior if you've haven't sustained at least a stab wound or two.

The British thinker Alan Watts said this about it: "To remain stable is to refrain from trying to separate yourself from a pain because you know that you cannot. Running away from fear is fear, fighting pain is pain, trying to be brave is being scared. If the mind is in pain, the mind is pain. The thinker has no other form than his thought. There is no escape."

No escape.

Maybe it was time to call the neurologist.

The minute I walk into the doctor's office I wonder if it's a real doctor's office. It has fake wood paneling on every single wall and a receptionist who looks like the woman who gets all the plastic surgery because she wants to be a human Barbie.

"Hi, can I help you?" The "hi" sounds like a "ha." I think she's from Texas.

I tell her I have an appointment with the neurologist. Ends up, he's the only doctor in this office. Briefly I wonder if the two of them are having a little workplace fling.

After I fill out paperwork (a task I have come to despise), she leads me to the exam room where I meet the man I've been dreading. Thankfully, he seems harmless, with his dark hair and big grin. If he dyed his eyebrows golden brown he'd look exactly like a sweet Rottweiler.

Seeing the neurologist is a completely different experience than seeing the regular doctor. There is no essential tremor talk. There is talk, however, of the possibility of Lyme disease (from a tick). Or Wilson's disease (a buildup of copper in the liver). Or a stroke (thanks to stress). Or a brain tumor (*yikes*). At this point I'm rooting for the stroke.

"Or," he says, "it could be Parkinson's disease."

No. That was my first thought. Just no. Like he asked me if I thought it was Parkinson's disease. No.

And then I thought, Oh, hell no.

And, That is not possible.

And, Don't be fucking ridiculous.

And, Dude, old people have Parkinson's disease.

"I'm only forty-two. Seriously?"

He was serious.

Aside from the fact that you have to be eighty, the extent of my knowledge on the subject was that Michael J. Fox sadly had it and that I didn't want it. I had no idea what it entailed, or that it had anything to do with dopamine, or why there was no cure. Although Mike seemed to be doing pretty well, which I knew because, coincidentally, I had just seen him on Oprah. He was still rich. His wife hadn't left him. *And* he did a ton of good for people. Yay for Alex P. Keaton.

However, I still didn't want it. That much hadn't changed.

"So what now?" I ask.

I was just kidding, he says.

"I'd recommend an MRI. As soon as possible." An MRI? Where they stick you in a machine and you get all claustrophobic?

"Is that really necessary?" I beg him with my eyes to say, Probably not.

"I'd like to rule anything else out."

Okay, then, be seein' ya!

Hoping to prevent a repeat of what happened after the last doctor, I get out of there as fast as I can. I'd almost be better off drinking than go through that again.

I also do not get the MRI as soon as possible.

Nor do I follow up with him.

Because that's just being *obsessive*.

And that is not healthy.

Besides, I can't afford it. Did I mention I have no health insurance? Of course I don't. I'm a bartender. A bartender who had to fork over $400 to be told I might have one of five horrible things wrong with me. If anything ends up seriously wrong, I'll just have to resort to voodoo.

If I was slightly scared before, now I'm that times ten. And completely unwilling to talk about it. Talking about it makes it real. And so does freaking out, and making desperate midnight phone calls, and posting sullen and cryptic stuff on Facebook. And to top it all off, this is what's happening right when I'm about to start a new yoga teacher training.

So here's a way to make a great first impression: you walk into a roomful of yoga teachers in this exact frame of mind, none of whom know you, who are gathered at the studio for the sole purpose of getting acquainted with the new trainees. And the reason they don't know you is because they teach in the mornings and you practice at night. Maybe it's a within-the-womb thing, but somehow it feels safer to practice at night.

Unfortunately for me, they do these things in the middle of the day when the studio is as bright as the goddamn sun. The thought of this stresses me to the bone until I'm practically ready to puke. But I rally. So what if I'm secretly having a nervous breakdown. *I'm gonna teach yoga.*

I drop Shamus off with my boyfriend Mauro. He tells me I look cute in my part-macrame gold silk dress I'm wearing, the one I'm hoping will serve as a decent enough distraction in case anything starts "going wrong."

Thanks babe! Wish me luck!

The whole way there I remind myself to sparkle. No one will want me around if they think I'm defective. Also, I have paid for this in full and there is no backing out.

I get there.

I march in.

Ready.

Confident.

Overcompensating.

And I leave in tears.

Nothing goes wrong or anything. In fact, it goes pretty well. Better than I could have hoped. I don't really even know why I'm crying.

I'm just so fucking tired.

I'm leading a double life. I'm John Wayne Gacy. I present myself in potentially awkward social situations as a laughing, colorful clown to gain your regard. If you ask friends and neighbors, they will tell you I'm "normal" and that I "keep to myself." Meanwhile, there's a crawlspace in the basement where I've buried my secrets. It's starting to get pretty crowded down there, but they are mine. And there they'll stay.

I get home from the thing and take a sad little nap. Later I go to work at the bar, where I pour eight thousand drinks I can't drink for all the nonshaky people. They thank me in cash tips. Then I get home at three in the morning, crawl into bed and will myself to pass out before the weight of the world squashes my soul like a tomato.

SUTURED #1: A BRIEF GUIDE THROUGH THE YOGA SUTRAS

Patanjali's Yoga Sutras are over two centuries old. And unless you have a PhD in philosophy, they can be awfully tricky to understand. Luckily, they're short and sweet, all 196 of them, and they come in four different parts. So let's go.

BOOK ONE

PORTION ON CONTEMPLATION

1. Let's do it. Right now. Hold your arms high and clap your hands once. That is the sound of *now*. And now's the time for yoga.

2. Yoga is the stoppage of every little annoying, petty, distracting, or otherwise flustering thought that might occur to you in this life.

3. And when those thoughts do stop, you'll be totally chill.

4. Otherwise, you are doomed to walk the Earth operating under the false assumption that the real you has anything to do with the you that's just a bunch of cells that happen to be

Hidden

stuck together.

5. You will also vacillate between thinking you suck and not thinking you suck.

6. There are five ways you'll come to the above conclusions: by having awareness of what's right in front of you (correct knowledge), by having zero awareness of what's right in front of you (illusion), by seeing something other than what's right in front of you (delusion), basically by being unconscious (sleep), or by conjuring up old, subconscious images that have nothing to do with anything (memory).

7. If you can see it, infer it, or read it from a reliable source, then you're probably okay.

8. But one day you might spot a mole on your body you'd never seen before and assume you are dying. And it might not even be a mole. It could just be dirt. So now you're just making stuff up.

9. Or you'll misconstrue something that may have been totally innocent. *Debbie just said hi to me. It was a weird hi. I'm pretty sure Debbie hates me.*

10. At night you'll go to sleep, which is basically the thought of having no thought.

11. Then one day, you might remember some random moment from your past, and you'll let it ruin your whole day.

12. Then you'll go off to yoga and be all, *whatever.*

13. But if you really want it to stop (and you do), half-assing it ain't gonna work. Neither will doing yoga every once in a while, which doesn't even constitute a "practice." That's more like a dabble.

14. So go for it. Do yoga and sit in meditation and contemplate your head off. Give it all you got. Turn the TV off and ignore the phone. I guarantee you will not miss any texts more important than this.

15. Nonattachment is the way to go. Not to be confused with indifference, which is a sign of depression. And being a sociopath. Nonattachment is more like, *Hey man, no worries.*

16. Then there's Supreme nonattachment. It's nonattachment, but supersized.

17. The only thing now that exists is existence. Awareness aware of awareness. You-ness.

18. …Until this moment: you're deep in meditation. And maybe you're feeling a little hungry, so you start thinking about where you might want to eat after this. And how they have yummy garden burgers at the one place next to that bar where you have to walk downstairs like they did in *Cheers.* Now you're thinking about that one episode of *Cheers* where Sam loses his lucky bottle cap and almost starts drinking again. And whatever happened to Shelley Long? And how you forgot to call your friend Shelley back, and she's probably pissed, and god, people get pissed easily. And on and on.

19. Then you'll have to come back in your next life and try

again. Luckily, your progress goes with you. Like rollover minutes.

20. You might also start to notice how much easier other people seem to have it. *Why's Debbie so fucking happy. It's so annoying.* Have faith, baby. Don't give up. You got this.

21. They'll be eating your dust soon anyway. That's how fast this thing moves. It's the cheetah of wisdom traditions.

22. But it's up to you, and you alone. No one's making you do this. So go big.

23. This is the part of the story where you might be, say, wandering across a desert landscape looking for your runaway droid when an enlightened being with a funky name shows up to blow your mind about what the Force is all about. Only here it's a concept: *Ishvara Pranidhana,* or Surrender to an Unchanging Reality.

24. Also known as the Ultimate Truth, *Ishvara* is an entity that is way bigger than all of us and has none of the aforementioned issues. Some call it God.

25. Ishvara knows everything.

26. Ishvara knows everything because it came before everything else came.

27. You can go ahead and call Ishvara by its more common name: OM.

28. Say it out loud. Say it a lot. In truth, you're saying it right

now anyway, because we are all made of vibration. Nothing is at rest. Everything is moving, spinning, radiating, mostly in space, creating ripples in the ocean of you. And the sound of it is OM.

29. Awesome. It's all gonna be okay!

30. Wait, what's that? An obstacle? Yup. Or nine, to be exact. They are: Physical Illness, Lack of Enthusiasm, Doubt, Carelessness, Laziness, Overindulging in Crappy Stuff, Distorted Perception, Failure to Find a Footing, and Instability to Maintain Progress.

31. I'd tell you not to despair, but you will. The minute one of these obstacles comes up you'll get all upset, and depressed, and you won't be able to sleep, and it'll all feel out of control.

32. But stay focused. Pace yourself, rabbit. The princess still needs saving.

33. And remember to not be an asshole just because things might not be going your way. No one will want to hang out with you. Be sweet. Give that hungry guy over there something to eat. Scream with joy when good things happen to people. Ignore all the rest.

34. And if you're really spun, do this: take a slow breath in, then a slow breath out, and then hold it there. Do this a few times.

35. Or spend a few minutes and sit there concentrating on one thing, and only one thing. Trip out on the tip of your nose.

36. ...Or a light, a brilliant light deep inside you, not like a strobe but more like a glow.

37. ...Or your heart. Your beautiful, open heart. There's love there.

38. ...Or a dream you may have had. Dreams are your subconscious trying to tell you something you may be missing.

39. ...Or anything you want. Something beautiful. I know you can think of something beautiful.

40. Soon enough you'll be vibrating all the way from the most infinitesimal part of your being—and who knows how small that really is, because they keep finding things, like planets and quarks—to the outer edges of the universe. Not that there are edges. I'm pretty sure it just keeps going.

41. Then nothing else will matter. And you'll be all, *Oh, hey, that wasn't so hard after all.*

42. But we are very, very good at confusing ourselves.

43. So forget everything you think you know.

44. ...Because it's screwing you all up.

45. Pretty soon your mind will wander less and less. The gods will be proud of you.

46. But stop asking if you're there yet, because the answer will be the same as when you asked me ten minutes ago: almost.

47. The good news is, you're getting to know the *real* you.

48. That's the you deep down inside.

49. Your horoscope will not reveal this you. Self-help books will not reveal this you. That wannabe guru on Hollywood Boulevard love-bombing you with empty words will not reveal this you.

50. And once you get to know the real you, there ain't no turnin' back. You are a cucumber that has turned into a pickle.

51. Way to go. We're moving in the right direction here. And we're gonna keep going until we're in sync with everything. What else do you have to do?

Only after disaster can we be resurrected. It's only after you've lost everything that you're free to do anything. Nothing is static, everything is evolving, everything is falling apart.

—CHUCK PALAHNIUK,

Fight Club

FOUR

DIAGNOSED

Take a minute, right now, and think about the second worst moment of your life. Not the worst moment—I don't want you getting all upset. Try to think about number two-ish. Or whatever. It's up to you.

Now think about what happened. Think about everything, what day of the week it was, and where you were, and what you might have been wearing, and who you were with, and if it was an equally bad moment for them too, and whether or not you saw this moment coming or it slammed you out of nowhere, and what happened afterward, and then ask yourself this: Did you respond to that moment at all the way you thought you would?

I'm thinking of a Monday. I'm in a doctor's office in Beverly Hills. I'm wearing jeans that probably could be a little less rippy, a black tank top under a black jacket made of corduroy and pleather and my studded peace-sign belt. I'm alone, unless you count the doctor, who (unlike myself) is probably just having a regular moment because he's just at work. No, I did not see it coming. (Maybe a little.) And later I'll go to the mall with my boyfriend for cinnamon lollipops.

My response was way off.

Dr. Bowen is neurologist #2. I'm getting a second opinion today on the second opinion. After neurologist #1 had the audacity to tell me I might have Parkinson's, I decided he was full of shit and that I never, ever wanted to see him again. Then I threw his card away and completely forgot his name. (Which is exactly what happens when you have Parkinson's. I still have no idea what that guy's name was.) Also, there was all that talk of MRIs and blood tests, and quite frankly I just wasn't up for it. Not while I had teacher training.

Somehow, I got through it. Twelve Friday nights of yoga philosophy, twelve Saturdays and Sundays of study/practice/teaching, and twelve weeks desperately trying to appear not sickly. And since working nights in a bar makes you kind of look (and sound) a little sickly during the day anyway, this ended up being double the effort. But the great thing about teacher trainings is you do a ton of yoga, and when you're not doing yoga you're assisting teaching yoga, and when you're not doing either one of those you're thinking about yoga, and with all that going on I really had no time to get to the bottom of things even though yoga teachers are definitely *not* supposed to look sickly. They're supposed to be a triple swirl of health and pluck and able-bodiedness. They're supposed to radiate with the light of a thousand suns.

Me, I radiate with something else. And it's really starting to piss me off.

The evil thing inside me (which is now what I'm

calling it) isn't going away. I now know what it feels like to be stalked. It's still very slight, but it's there, under my skin, munching away on my last nerve and fucking up my life. And it's relentless. It's annoying. It's Glenn Close in *Fatal Attraction* and it refuses to be ignored.

Never in my life did I have a better reason to sit at home and be in a bad mood. And believe me, I wanted to. I wanted to build an imaginary wall around me and be my own country. Just me and Shamus. No ins and outs. But I'd also just spent three months doing all that yoga, and yoga has a way of ruining your bad mood in the exact same way AA ruins your drinking. It's just not fun anymore once you know you have an out.

Convincing myself to go to the doctor at this point wasn't hard. Part of it was morbid curiosity. For all I knew still I could have had a brain tumor, which is the other thing the last guy said. I'm not a doctor but I don't think you should ignore tumors of any kind, and especially not ones in your head. Or maybe it was something else entirely. I've seen enough episodes of *House* to know there are plenty of obscure and totally curable diseases out there, and I very well could have had one of them. *This girl doesn't have a neurological condition. She has a worm infestation in her spinal column. Let's give her a pill that'll fix her right up.*

It *was* hard, however, to get an appointment at a decent

hour. So by the time I screech into the parking lot of the doctor's office at ten after eight in the morning, I'm already late. Thirty minutes late, if you include the whole "please arrive twenty minutes early for your appointment" thing. Which is now shot.

(It's possible I didn't leave on time. And that I stopped at Starbucks. And lingered.)

I run past a valet who wants to know how long I'll be. "Not long," I call back, hoping he'll assume I'm a messenger and not a patient. I then take the elevator to the sixth floor, which dumps me out into the longest hallway ever. Dr. Bowen's office is at the end.

This feels like a slight error in judgment. If you're someone like a neurologist or a dentist or anyone else people aren't that stoked to see, don't ever put your office far away from the elevator. This gives a person time to think. And what I'm thinking is I'm about to walk into a room likely filled with Parkinson's people, all of them in wheelchairs, shaking like frightened Chihuahuas, staring catatonically at their caregivers who are wiping the person's drool off their own shoes. And if that's what's going on in there I might have to bail on this whole thing and reschedule from the hallway. I could barely watch the movie *Awakenings*. Although that was different. I think.

I crack open the door. There's no one in there but

empty furniture and a yawning receptionist. *Phew*.

"Hi, can I help you?"

"Hi, I have an appointment with Dr. Bowen."

"And your name?"

I tell her it's Anne, wishing it wasn't. And not because I never liked it. It's just something like this would never happen to a Paris. Or a Tallulah. I should really think about using an alias from now on.

The receptionist tells me I'm fifteen minutes late. I whip out the L.A. excuse. "Yeah….Traffic."

There was no traffic. I live less than five miles away from there. And shaming the potentially sick-in-the-brain person who has to come see the neurologist in the first place is not cool, but whatever. Secretly I'm hoping she'll just send me home. Instead she hands me paperwork to be filled out. "Front and back, please."

Neurology paperwork is like regular doctor paperwork but with mysterious questions interspersed that make you wonder. Am I right handed, left handed, or ambidextrous? (Right handed ✓) Why do you need to see a neurology specialist? (My left hand has been shaking.) Have you ever seen a neurologist? (Yes ✓) What was the diagnosis? (There's no box for "I blew the whole thing off" so I leave it blank.) Have you experienced daily vomiting for the last two days or longer? (Uh, no ✓) Have you had any hospitalizations or operations? (No ✓) Have you had any blood transfusions? (No ✓) Did you grow up on a farm or drink well water growing up? (Huh? No ✓)

The next part is the longest list of possible symptoms imaginable for any condition, some of which I've never heard of. Am I supposed to know if I have ataxia? Or polyneuropathy? And how does one know if they have enlarged nodes? There's also drooling, choking, blurred vision, chills, irregular heartbeat, inability to smell, ringing in the ears, double vision, convulsions, seizures, and on and on.

Two things get checked: dizziness and clumsiness. There is nothing new about either one of them. So now I'm worried I might have something wrong that's been going on for longer than I thought, and that whatever it was I probably should have just faced the music and taken care of it already and saved myself from all the nonsense I'd been putting myself through, and that now I may have reached the stage when it was "too late."

What happened to Anne? I heard she keeled over dead. Yeah. She refused to get that tremor looked at. She waited way too long.

This may have been the moment I realized how overwhelmed I really was. I imagine it's how an ant must feel when they see a shoe coming. And in a matter of minutes I'd be seeing the doctor, and I had no idea what I'd do if he had bad news, except maybe leave and go *Thelma and Louise*-it off a cliff. Or self-implode on the spot. *Kablooey*. Blood and guts everywhere. Then I'd have no choice but to scrape myself off the walls, go home, and get back to work on that imaginary wall.

But here's the sneaky thing about yoga. Not sneaky like, *I'm gonna shank you the second you turn around*, but more like, *Silly mortal. Watch and learn*.

Joseph Campbell wrote a book called *Myths to Live By*. And in this book, there is a chapter where he compares what he calls the "LSD phenomenon" to yoga. Both, he said, produce a similar experience of psychosis. Both are a break from the world, a plunge into a deep inward sea, an "intentionally achieved schizophrenia." Because here's what he said the pattern of a schizophrenic breakdown looks like: first, there's a separation from what would be considered your normal life. Then you retreat into what we think of as the soul and have all kinds of terrifying experiences with what scares you. Confronting these things gives you new courage and, if you're fortunate enough, you'll come back to a life of harmony. Because that's what the schizophrenic is really doing—trying to achieve contact with a part of themselves they perceive to be missing so they can regain a sense of integration and feel normal again.

Acid. Yoga. Take your pick. But know what Joseph Campbell said was the important difference: The LSD guy will enter the mystical waters of that inner sea "unprepared, unguided, and ungifted, has fallen or has intentionally plunged, and is drowning." And the yogi will dive into that same sea and instinctually know how to swim.

I'm halfway through a magazine article about aneurysms when they summon me into the exam room. It's cold and white, like the inside of an igloo. Outside the window I can see the tops of palm trees and all I want to do is go sit on one.

The doctor comes in. "Hi, Anne, I'm Dr. Bowen."

Dr. Bowen immediately strikes me as the sweet and boring type. He is the exact guy who would come in second on *The Bachelor*, get his own season, spend four months in a lackluster relationship with a pharmaceutical salesgirl from Kentucky, and, ultimately, never find love. But you root for him anyway.

He sits down on his wheeled stool. "So tell me what's going on."

I tell him the whole story. When it all started, what it's like now, blah blah blah. He listens intently. It's actually nice. I never talk about it.

Once he knows more about my situation than any other person on the planet, which is four minutes later, he proceeds to give me a series of tests just like when you get pulled over for a DUI.

"Okay, Anne, I want you to stand up and touch your nose for me, one finger at a time."

I do it.

"Now tap your thumb and forefinger together on both hands."

I do that too. Handily.

"Now I'm going to give you three words to remember, and in a minute I'm going to ask you to repeat them. Orange. Pencil. Cat."

Got it.

"Now say the alphabet backwards."

"Z Y X W V U T S R Q… P? Yeah, P O N M L K… J! I H G F E D C B A."

"Great. Now can you walk in a straight line for me?"

I do it. This is actually kind of fun.

"And can you tell me the three words?

"Orange. Pencil. Cat."

Nailed it.

"Now hold out your right arm and resist me as I push it down."

I do it and it goes nowhere because I'm strong.

"And now your left."

I do it and it goes halfway down. A little more, actually. Like a sad flagpole.

There's a pause.

Maybe he didn't just see that.

Oh, but he did.

Not only did he see it, but he's been taking notes this whole time. But we continue anyway, like it didn't happen, which is fine with me. "Okay, Anne, hold out both arms for me now, and make fists then open your fingers wide as quick as you can."

I do it. The left one is definitely slower than the right.

"And the three words again are…?"

"Orange. Pencil. Cat."

At this point I'm wondering if this is really what they teach in medical school and if we could have done this over Skype. It couldn't possibly be definitive of anything. So what if one of my arms was weaker than the other? I could've slept on it wrong. That alone could've brought down my whole score, unless this was a pass/fail thing. He didn't say.

"Anne, I think you have Parkinson's disease."

Diagnosed

And, fail.

He thinks I have Parkinson's disease.

HE THINKS I HAVE MUTHA EFFING PARKINSON'S DISEASE.

Now, I don't know if anyone's ever told you they think you have Parkinson's disease, but speaking of schizophrenia, maybe you'll understand what happens next: just for a moment, my mind splits into five minds, all of which have their own different personalities that are all aspects of me, and all five of those parts of me shoot out of the gate and react in five completely different ways in a sudden race to see who will dominate.

Will it be the seventeen year old in me who wants to light a cigarette and blow smoke in his face?

The adult in me who wants to hear him out?

The writer in me who wishes I was taping this?

Someone else, I'm not sure who, who just wants to laugh?

Or the barefoot hippie chick in me who is meditating and strangely not at all bothered?

Final score: tied.

Dr. Bowen, who I imagine probably hates these moments, is kind of just sitting there staring at me. In a way I almost feel worse for him. Except I'm sure if he ever does go on *The Bachelor* he can tell sad stories about telling people they have Parkinson's and girls will love it.

"How do you know?" I finally utter.

"Well, your symptoms are consistent with Parkinson's," he says. "But we can never know for sure unless they do an autopsy." Meaning, dead. Awesome.

I have no clue what else to ask. I definitely don't want any similar answers to the last one. So I look out the window at the palm trees, only they're not so much palm trees now as they are witnesses, seers of one of the weirdest moments of my life as it unfolded.

"Look, I know a group..." Dr. Bowen is trying to be helpful. "It's a support group for young people with Parkinson's. One guy in the group is an FBI agent."

If he thinks I care to sit in a group of strangers discussing the situation, he obviously doesn't know me. I don't care how cool there are.

"I really don't think I'm ready for that."

He stabs a pamphlet at me anyway. "I have a number of young patients who find the groups really helpful."

I bet you do. And I'm sure a number of people found Jim Jones and the People's Temple really helpful.

This, I keep to myself. I wouldn't want him writing any derogatory comments in my file, like "patient is not receptive to simple suggestion. I'd put her chances of being happy at about one out of forty."

I tell him I'll think about it. And then I wonder how many people say that.

I leave with a handful of dopamine pills and walk the long ass hallway back to the elevator. It takes me down to my car where I see the same valet who charges me $15 to park, which seems incredibly lame under the circumstances, but whatever.

Five minutes later, I'm back on the road. The whole thing is literally in my rearview mirror.

And that was the beginning of what should have been the worst day ever. The day I should have shattered into a million pieces. But I'm kind of calm, and maybe a little relieved. I was way more freaked out after I saw the other two doctors, and all they did was suggest I *might* have a neurological problem of some sort, but the suggestion of it ended up being far worse than actually hearing it, which wasn't all that fantastic either, but at least I'm still intact. And in a way, that's the most shocking thing of all. *The lack of shock.* Which might make it sound like I actually *am* in shock, which may have been the case had I not just been through that teacher training, when over and over we heard the same words from K. Pattabhi Jois: *practice, and all is coming.*

Practice, and what should be one of the worst days of your life might not be.

Practice, and you won't feel like losing your mind when you get told you have a fucking horrible disease.

Practice, and you'll know there's no scary monster on the wing of the plane.

Practice, and you'll experience an inordinate amount of gratitude for your life and everything in it.

Practice, and you might change your mind tomorrow and decide you hate everyone.

Practice, and you'll change it back again the next day.

Practice, and you won't end up drowning in the mystical waters of that inner sea.

I drive straight to Mauro's house. He's barely awake, so I put a pot of coffee on and tell him the whole story, fully expecting him to regret ever meeting me and say maybe it's time we see other people. Instead he tells me four hundred times in a row how much he loves me and that he always will no matter what.

Later we go to the mall. And the whole day ends with cinnamon lollipops.

We're freaks, that's all. Those two bastards got us nice and early and made us into freaks with freakish standards, that's all. We're the tattooed lady, and we're never going to have a minute's peace, the rest of our lives, until everybody else is tattooed, too.

—J.D. SALINGER

FIVE

FREAKY

I'm in my first teaching audition, four minutes to go, trying to decide if I should lie my way out of there. The tremor is acting up, and at the worst possible moment. But I can't stand liars, mostly because lying in general is just immature, and the thought of becoming someone I would normally not be able to stand in a matter of minutes is almost as bothersome as my stupid tremor hand.

(I'm not supposed to do that. "Don't hate the disease," my neurologist encourages me. "Find a fun way to fit it into the conversation, like, *Oh, look at that, I spilled coffee all over myself. It's just the ol' Parkinson's! No big deal, this shirt's washable!* You see?" Yeah. I do see. And I encourage myself to not tell him to go fuck himself.)

The hour doesn't help. I had to get up at the crack of dawn this morning to meet up with Drorit, the studio owner at 7:30, which means I got about four hours of sleep. And somehow getting four hours of sleep is almost worse than if you've never slept at all. I probably should have just stayed up.

These are not the bartending hours I'm used to. This is not the work environment I'm used to. The bar is all murky lighting and deafening loud music, not morning sun and chirping birds. There I can hide under fedora hats and a pound and a half of eyeliner, obscuring the horror of the fact that I'm not like everyone else and I can't even have one drink to ease my nerves about the situation. Not that it would make anything better. I don't even want to drink, but I almost want to want to. It would be so easy, at least for a minute there until I remember, *oh yeah, I don't drink because I crash cars and throw up in public. And hello, jail? Remember jail?*

Jail. Parkinson's disease. Same thing. And they both suck.

Then there's the medication. Dopamine meds are weird and kind of hellish. They make you dizzy and forgetful and wide awake all at the same time. I find myself hurriedly stumbling into walls while trying to remember what day it is. I hit my anklebone a lot. I lose track of where my car is in crowded parking structures. Don't ask me what I ate for lunch yesterday. No clue.

No one warns you about this. I was told, however, to watch out for a gambling addiction to develop and that I should steer clear of Vegas. Apparently all that extra dopamine makes you compulsive and reckless. This is the number one side effect. So on top of everything else, now I have to worry about ending up sick and penniless in the desert after losing everything at the blackjack table. Or learn how to count cards. Might as well put all that compulsiveness to good use.

So the plan this morning was to show up and try to act

normal. Like I'm the healthiest human being in the world. Fit as a fiddle and Zen as fuck. Like I didn't have Parkinson's at all. None of that "fitting it into the conversation" crap, no *hey, just so you know….*

I could do it. *Pfft.* I did it every single day.

I get there at 7:30. Early. So far so good. Drorit arrives right after me. She is lovely. The studio is beautiful and cozy. We chat, we do a little yoga, and things go so well, I decide to stay for her 9:00 a.m. class. It's going great. What was I so worried about?

First mistake: lingering too long in one place. Always keep moving. Like a wolf.

No, first mistake: not walking in with a fiberglass cast on and some kind of story about how I broke my arm, which I realize would have called more attention to my hand but at least the shaking would have been theoretically trapped.

Once things get flowing I'm actually feeling amazing. Sometimes I forget how good it feels to do yoga first thing in the morning. Sometimes I wish I could forget a lot of things.

"Inhale, and reach your arms high for Warrior One," Drorit is saying. "Exhale, open up for Warrior Two…." I'm in the zone. "And moving into Half Moon…."

And then it starts happening. I can feel it. I feel it the way you feel a fly on your skin.

Things may have all gone downhill from there.

Under different circumstances, but definitely not under these circumstances, I'd almost respect its cunning. There's something very sharklike about it. Out of nowhere: DANGER. And as we all know from *Jaws*, when a shark appears the last thing you want to do is make a big splashy fuss or you'll end up getting chomped. So in an effort to not panic, which I'm here to tell you does make things much worse—at least with Parkinson's, and apparently with sharks—I fix my gaze on the wall, the color of cobalt blue. Or is it Caribbean blue? Or navy? Whatever. I believe it is supposed to be a soothing blue, but it definitely isn't. It's hateful. And so is the fuckhead who said it was supposed to be soothing in the first place. I've seriously never hated a color so much in my life. *It failed me.*

Stupid blue. Fucking tremor hand.

Since it's nearly impossible at this point to find a meat cleaver in the immediate vicinity and chop off my hand without being noticed, I close my eyes and try to remember every breathing trick I've ever learned. *Inhale for ten.... Hold your breath....* Exhale for 10.... Wait. Didn't I see a 7-Eleven across the street? Yes! They probably had sharp instruments for sale! Hopefully the blood wouldn't stain the bamboo floors too much, and in my defense I could always blame the whole thing on Endorphin Rush

Syndrome (which I just made up).

Second mistake: not bringing a meat cleaver.

Meanwhile, unlike my blood pressure, time has managed to slow down to a crawl. By now I feel like it should be tomorrow. I imagine this must be how it feels to get shot and watch the life drain out of you. This is when I start thinking about lying.

I could fake a stomachache, which would not be difficult.

Or I could act like I forgot I had to be somewhere, at 10:16 on a Tuesday morning.

Or I could create a diversion. *Earthquake. Fire. Land shark.*

Third mistake: not thinking of a good enough lie.

I start wondering what the other fifteen or so people in the room are thinking about. Mundane shit, probably. No one else seems to be having a Parkinson's attack or cursing the blue walls. I certainly don't see "crisis" written on anybody else's face. They're in Pigeon Pose. After class I'm sure they're probably headed to the market for oatmeal or lemons or soap. Or maybe they have to meet up with the cable guy. Or they'll go to the pressed juice place for a tasty wheatgrass shot. Tuesday stuff. Who knows? Maybe someone will go home to find a note: *Gwen, I'm leaving you. I want a divorce. Keep the Land Rover.*

Yoga rooms are full of secrets. Honestly, I'm surprised you don't see more people flipping out. It may seem like the exact wrong place, like being drunk in an AA meeting, which I've actually seen quite a bit of and hey, hats off for honesty.

Maybe it was time for me to be honest too. *I'm sorry, Drorit, but I can't do this. I've managed to hide it up until now, but my hand is shaking and you're going to find out I have Parkinson's Disease. They tell me I may have brought it on myself by early drug and alcohol abuse. Or too many Ding Dongs. No one knows. My point is, I probably should have thought this through and opted to blow it off, stay at home safely in bed watching a fantastically insipid* Three's Company *marathon and avoid the entire planet.*

P.S. If you happen to have a meat cleaver, I could really use it to chop my hand off. I won't blame you if you don't end up hiring me. And sorry about the floors.

I'm in hell. I'm separate from everyone and everything. I'm John Travolta in *The Boy in the Plastic Bubble*.

I had never felt less like myself. And that's the worst feeling in the world.

I remember walking into a mall once when I was three days sober. Somebody should've stopped me, or at least loaned me a second brain for the time being. Sometimes you need it. Three days into sobriety is one of them. On day one, you're just hungover. Day two, you're still a little fuzzy. By day three, you wake up feeling like the biggest loser ever. And everyone knows it.

They can all tell, I thought as I made my way through the bustling food court. They all know what a fuckup I am. Any minute they're going to rise up and start throwing stones at me. I felt like Hester Prynne with her scarlet letter. A for Alcoholic.

There's a line in Lisa Lowry's book *The Giver*: "I feel sorry for anyone who is in a place where he feels strange and stupid." For the longest time, I was sure I could never feel any more strange or stupid than I did that day in the mall. But it was nothing compared to what I felt in that yoga class.

Imagine your worst problem. Make it a really awful one, assuming you have a really awful one. Even a mediocre one will do. Maybe you have an illness or a secret shame, something that may or may not be your fault. Something you've strategically hidden underneath the bed with the broken hangers and other crap you haven't bothered throwing away. Something you're completely positive that, if you told your best friend the truth about, they'd never stop screaming. Take a minute if you need. I can wait.

Ready? Now take a Sharpie and write it across your forehead. Use huge block letters. If it's in capitals, it'll be like you're yelling. One or two exclamation points might also drive it home. Go to work, go to yoga, go to Disneyland. Your annoying friends will tell you, *There's nothing to be afraid of. Everyone will be cool.* Here's my other fave: *You should really think about being more open with people about it.* Which is terrible advice, by the way. Same with, "Do the thing you're most afraid of." Okay. I'll tell people what's going on if you lick a trash can.

Having Parkinson's is like having a secret that everyone knows, which I realize doesn't make it much of a secret, but still. The thing is, they can't quite put their finger on it.

Your hand is shaking.... Are you OK?

Why are you sitting on your hand?

Why did you leave yoga class without one word?

There's just no good answer for any of that. I guess I could slam my head against the wall over and over. That might work.

Sometimes it's almost funny. Funny ha-ha. Of course I woke up one day at forty-two years old with this shit. Of course this is my life. Maybe tomorrow I'll get hit by a bus!

Freaky

Then one day I'll be sitting around, not doing much, just flipping channels on TV, and something will come on about Muhammad Ali. "The Greatest." And there he'll be, the most badass athlete of the twentieth century, a heavyweight champion no less, stuck in a wheelchair. His body stiff. His head tremoring. And it'll hit me: *There's my future.*

What Muhammad Ali had was slightly different, but the symptoms are the same. Thanks to getting punched in the head too many times, Ali ended up with Parkinson's syndrome. Also called pugilistic brain syndrome. At least he had a decent story behind his Parkinson's. Ali *earned* his disorder. Where was my punch in the head? Where was my super fly nickname? My brother calls me Tater, which I love, but Tater has Parkinson's. And not the cool pugilistic Parkinson's. Good ol' fashioned, fucking neurodegenerative disease Parkinson's.

Parkinson's. God I hate that word.

"Well, you're lucky in one respect," my mother told me once. "You won't die from it." So it's non-deadly, but you can't get rid of it. I'm not sure that's a good thing. A million shitty things can happen that won't necessarily kill you. I knew someone who had shingles once and she said it was unbelievably painful. Someone else I used to know caught some weird virus and went suddenly blind. You can get the thing where you stop tasting food. Or chronic hiccups. A limb might get removed. Or a lung.

And what if my "luck" runs out? It can't last forever. I could end up with mercury poisoning or a fatal blood clot. My appendix could burst. Tell me if brain aneurysms hurt, because I swear I feel a slight pressure by my left ear. And come to think of it, that itchy spot by my shoulder blade? It's cancer.

The great thing is, if you spend long enough online, you can find a cure for anything. Imagine my optimism when I came across the Zapper. The Zapper is an electronic contraption that looks exactly like a Mattel Handheld Football Game with little metal rods attached. It promises to "kill parasites, viruses, bacteria, mold, and fungi" that create blockages in your system so you can't absorb vital nutrients. Apparently nothing survives this thing. At first I wasn't sure if it was bullshit or not, but it was cheap and supposedly harmless. I changed my mind after seeing actual photos of what the parasites look like when they slither out of a person. The Zapper is still in the box.

I pass manicure places and long to inhale the toxic fumes of nail lacquer because I've had to stop getting manicures. I also avoid most situations in which strangers show up and touch you, like massages and acupuncture. Correct me if I'm wrong, but I'm afraid one of those

Freaky

needles will poke me in the wrong area and send my energy further into whackville. I'm better off at home. You'd be amazed how much you can get done when you stay at home all the time. *Surprise, Honey! I dyed my hair blue today!*

You can find inspiration anywhere. This is why I own every single Rocky movie. *Rocky* knows how to take a punch, and go the distance. We could all learn from the Italian Stallion. Just hearing the *Rocky* theme brings tears to my eyes. Reading memoirs from drug-addicted rock stars can also be inspiring. Then you can say *well, it could be worse, at least I'm not wasted right now, like some people.* Then it backfires when I get to the end and I realize they're still rich and famous once they get sober, and I'm broke and sick. Screw you, Eric Clapton.

The other thing that has occurred to me is that an unknowable dark force is trying to keep me down because I am a genius. And that it must be the same force that got to Stephen Hawking. I read an article once about it. The theory is Stephen Hawking is so damn smart he was on the cusp of unraveling the secrets of the universe, but those secrets aren't necessarily *supposed* to be known, so this force was sent to swoop in and give him ALS when he was twenty-one years old. Obviously it didn't stop him, because then he wrote the book *A Brief History of Time* about black holes, and space, and the nature of the observable universe (which is one million miles and twenty-four zeros long). So remember that if something goes wrong. You too, could be a genius.

One day I got completely sick of myself and went off to yoga. It was not my most fantastic day. Afterward someone in class told someone else they had noticed my hand shaking and that I must have been hungover. I didn't know whether to laugh, cry, or stab him in the neck. *I'M TWENTY-FIVE YEARS SOBER, YA MOTHERFUCKER, AND I AM NOT HUNGOVER.*

Next time just kick me in the organs. Seriously. Or throw acid in my face. Or yank me by the hair, pull me down the stairs, and toss me into the alley with yesterday's trash. Then point your finger at me and chant the words "circus freak, circus freak" at the top of your lungs to the tune of "Ring around the Rosie." I'm quite sure it would hurt less.

This is when shunning the world becomes an option. Blowing off everything. Hiding. Finding a padded cell and someone to bring me food and important news updates. Or building myself a cabin in the middle of the forest and becoming a recluse. Or maybe I could cut a chunk of the world off, float away on it and live like the Little Prince. At least nobody would be around to say anything stupid.

Freaky

I think about meditating more. Or differently. I think about moving to the middle of nowhere in Oregon or Canada where the air is bound to be much cleaner. I think about running ten miles a day, but not in a circle—more like in one long continuous line as far as I can go. Like Forrest Gump. One time I read Parkinson's is in your blood, so I think of what would happen if I got all my blood replaced with better blood. I think about what you must be thinking. But mostly, I think about what it would be like to *not* think about it.

Later that week, I'm slinging drinks at the bar. It's a typical Friday night. Boozed up, tarted up, cross-dressing fedora'd party freaks are everywhere, covered head to toe in glitter, ready to disco down. Tattooed chicks channel Bette Page in their black leather getups and fishnet stockings. Leggy boys in corsets and vinyl pencil skirts teeter in their twelve-inch heels, spilling their martinis. I always thought if Mad Max and the Black Swan ever got it on, this is totally what their offspring would look like.

Welcome to Hollywood.

A short man resembling Danny DeVito sidles up to the bar wearing a 1950s slip dress and a pink turkey-feather boa. I know him. He comes every week. I make him the drink special, a Skinny Bitch. "Cheers, babe." We clink glasses. Me with my soda water, and Danny DeVito with his Skinny Bitch.

My friend "Julie" shows up. Julie has the longest getaway sticks I've ever seen, and in the highest stilettos. I adore her. I also happen to know she's a very successful movie producer in real life named Jimmy.

"Hey doll," Julie/Jimmy says. "Am I wearing too much Chanel No5?"

I love it when people call me doll. What an old-fashioned bunch they are. And yes, she is wearing too much Chanel No5. But I'm way more preoccupied with worry over her knee joints.

"Be careful in those things," I say with a wink. Like I wasn't inappropriately wearing six-inch-tall thigh-high leopard boots at a BBQ last weekend.

"Annie!" My friend Randy is there. I'm always glad to see Randy. He and I talk about quantum physics, Buddhism, our mutual love of Patti Smith, literature, everything. Randy had me read *The Hitchhiker's Guide to the Galaxy*, and from that, I give you this: "There is a theory which states that if ever anyone discovers exactly what the universe is for and why it is here, it will instantly disappear and be replaced by something even more bizarre and inexplicable. There is another theory which states that this has already happened."

Bizarre and inexplicable. It summed up my entire situation. Earlier that week I was with the neurologist discussing what to do about my dopamine deficiency, and now I'm pouring Skinny Bitches for men in drag.

And staring out at that crowd, I realized something else: they had each other. There was no "outside," no glass for anyone to press their hands and nose against, gazing in, longing for that kind of freedom and acknowledgement and maybe the permission to belong someplace, anyplace where their secret uniqueness would normally disqualify them from admittance. No one judged "Julie" for wearing stilettos or for not knowing the appropriate amount of perfume to apply. No one cared if Danny DeVito was in a dress. Danny DeVito was, in fact, a brilliant engineer who just earned a scholarship to MIT. He's probably building skyscrapers right now in Dubai.

The depressing fact is that isolation can actually kill you. Too much alone time screws with your hormones and weakens your immune system. You get depressed, you gain weight, your blood pressure rises and it all goes downhill from there. Tumors grow faster in lonely people. They have higher instances of heart disease, Alzheimer's, schizophrenia, suicide. Everything bad.

In the nineties, UCLA did a study on HIV-positive gay men. Ends up, the closeted men were more likely to develop full-blown AIDS and pass away earlier. Living with the pain and fear of possible rejection, along with the pressure of having to monitor every single thing they said and did, created a constant state of terror. This triggered their stress hormones—specifically, norepinephrine. The HIV virus can replicate itself three to ten times faster in an environment where norepinephrine is present. White blood cell counts rise. Their systems became unable to fight. Having to maintain their "false identity" had drained them.

It doesn't matter who you are. A pack of misfits. Men with HIV. A group of Civil War reenactors. Everyone needs a wolf pack.

Wolves are highly social animals. They live and hunt in packs. It's their extended family. They're known to demonstrate deep affection for each other and may even sacrifice themselves to protect their family unit.

A wolf that has been driven from the pack or has left on its own is called a lone wolf. A lone wolf will die when it can't catch enough food by itself and when it doesn't have the protection of a pack. It avoids contact with others and rarely howls.

This is the saddest thing I've ever heard.

I don't want to hide. I don't want to be alone. I don't want to wander off into the desert in shame and die and become vulture food. Or end up keeling over just because I'm too self-conscious to leave the house. Cause of death: *unnecessary loneliness.*

I want to belong. Belonging makes things okay, and I want to be okay. I just want to be okay. And then I want to howl about it.

The Yoga Sutras say, "The cause of *bandha* and *moksha* (bondage and liberation) is our own minds. If we think we are bound, we are bound. If we think we are liberated, we are liberated. It is only when we transcend the mind that we are free from all these troubles."

Enough was enough. I knew what I had to do. So one day I spilled my guts out in an email to the one person I knew who wouldn't be weird, my teacher Jenny. My purple-haired, tattooed yoga teacher Jenny. If you saw her on the street, you'd think punk rocker. To know her is to think, *creature of uncommon specialness.* And she has no idea how grateful I am for her.

-----Original Message-----
From: Anne Clendening
To: Jenny Brill
Sent: Thu, Aug 4, 2011 6:13 PM
Subject: Need some advice. From YOU.

Dear Jenny,

This is going to seem totally out of the blue, but I think you're the person to come to. I saw a neurologist and it ends up I have Parkinson's. He put me on dopamine which makes me crazy dizzy. All I want is to go to yoga. And teach. As you may guess this isn't easy. I walk around in constant terror. As I'm writing this I'm about to start sobbing. I'm having a hard time showing up to class, but I know I need it now more than ever. Thanks Jenny, and please keep this between us :-) I just needed to vent. I appreciate any words of wisdom you can give me. Thanks, you're the best.

Love ya <3 Annie

From: Jenny Brill
To: Anne Clendening
Sent: Fri, Aug 5, 2011 9:23 AM
Subject: Re: Need some advice. From YOU.

First of all, I'm here for you no matter what. Second of all, I do agree that now more than ever you need your yoga. It's what gets us crazies through the rough times. And listen up my love—yoga can mean so many things in life. Let's not forget that the postures are but one small part of the bigger picture that yoga is! Meditation is also yoga, walking is yoga, stretching is yoga, it's all the intention behind it. You need to get into your body and use what's going on to propel you forward however you can. You will get jobs because you are a fucking kick-ass teacher. Allow this to be a turning point and you can say one day, "Remember when I got diagnosed and everything changed and I started teaching a whole bunch?"

She was right. About all of it. And I got that teaching job I went out for. I'd say I got two or three solid days of liberation after that, until I found out what it was really like to teach.

Ring the bells (ring the bells) that still can ring
Forget your perfect offering
There is a crack in everything (there is a crack in everything)
That's how the light gets in

—LEONARD COHEN, *Anthem*

SIX

UNBROKEN

It's three months later. I have not exploded yet. Close. I am, however, starting to run out of patience.

Secretly I was hoping this thing would just peter out on its own at some stage, but that doesn't seem to be happening any time soon and frankly, I'm a little surprised. I guess I wasn't listening on Parkinson's orientation day when they said the words *progressive* and *incurable*. I do believe the moment those words slither into your reality is the day you know you're doomed. Same with *chronic*. They're the verbal equivalent of being jumped into a gang you don't want to be in. Those words are way bigger than they sound. And way darker.

Telling Jenny definitely lifted a little bit of the burden. Thank god for email. I never could have done it in person. And things had gotten so intense I'd forgotten what it was like to let someone be there for me, someone besides Mauro, but we live together now, so he pretty much has no choice.

"You're beautiful," he'll say every morning.

You're just saying that, I'll reply.

"You are. You're beautiful."

He is beautiful.

Unfortunately, Jenny is only one person. There are billions of others out there and I know at least a thousand of them. Some of them even come to my yoga class which, like myself, may have gone a little off the rails.

Yes, there will be inappropriately loud music tonight. I'm thinking Metallica. And no, we are not working on stillness, we are movingmovingmoving. And did I keep you in Down Dog a little too long? That's because I can't remember for the life of me what we did on the first side and I needed time to think. Oh, and sorry I was late. I was at the neurologist.

The stress of teaching was insane. I came to dread it. You literally could have pulled a gun on me and I would have been less panic stricken. And the panic was there, staring me in the face, all the time, like I had a hoodie on backwards and I couldn't get it off.

Yup. I'm a yoga teacher with fear in my bones and dread in my heart. You can email the management for refunds.

(Side note: my friend Gretchen ended up saying that the Metallica class was the most fun one ever. So maybe there really is something out there for everyone.)

Right around then I'd also managed to develop an irrational resentment against time, which had screwed me, because who comes down with a problem like this the minute they start teaching yoga unless maybe they'd murdered someone in their last life. It was the only feasible explanation for something I found completely unacceptable, and also maybe the reason why I'd been having visions of straight up killing it. I wanted to put an end to its miserable reign, which was what—almost two years by then? I wanted to go *Kill Bill* on it with my yellow jumpsuit on and a Hanzo sword in my hand and get my stab on. Or chop. Whatever it was. Maybe then I wouldn't feel like such an aberration, an "accidental guest in this dreadful body," to use a line from the tortured soul Anna Akhmatova. And why rely on everything you ever learned about yourself in yoga when you can be sitting around reading Russian poetry about suffering and despair. As you can see it's working out *extremely* well. Just like everything else I've tried.

First, there was Bowen therapy. Bowen therapy is like a massage, but not. A person will use the slightest pressure imaginable to move specific areas of soft tissue around to stimulate your nerve passages and give your whacked out body a chance to calm down. This takes like, a second. Then they leave you alone for two minutes. They do this over and over for an hour and you fall into an amazingly deep sleep. Afterward you wake up feeling totally refreshed and a little drugged. I could have done it every day, but Bowen therapy costs a lot, and I needed money for stuff like food and rent.

Next there were the liquid something-or-other drops

I ordered from Australia. The theory behind the drops is you're dehydrated and you don't know it. This goes for everyone. So the drops make you thirsty and help your cells absorb water, giving you more energy, hydrating your organs and restoring your long lost balance. *Biofeedback studies have shown it.* Also, they're not even available here, so I knew it must be really good shit. For $95, they better be. And who needs FDA approval?

The day the Australia box comes, I immediately open it and inspect the tiny bottle. The label reads, "All Natural & Infused with Herbal Essences." I have no idea what this means, but it sounds very healthy. So three times a day I'll put five–seven drops of it in the recommended mix of forty percent juice/sixty percent water and drink it from something nonplastic and see how it goes.

My friend Justine has been warning me about plastic for years. "You need to get it out of your house," she said once. "All of it."

I asked her how that was possible. Only everything has plastic in it.

"You just do it. It's killing all of us. That, and antiperspirants."

I don't know how I'm supposed to feel about these kinds of statements. But if I ever move to a deserted island, I'm taking Justine with me. She's my Earth Child friend.

One day Justine came over with a jar of powdered "food" for me to try called *Mucuna pruriens. Mucuna pruriens* supposedly enhances brain function, soothes your nervous system, and makes you feel good. But it looked and smelled like dirt, so I put it up on a shelf, right next to the drops which didn't do anything, and forgot all about both of them.

Then there was the day I spent at the IV clinic. I had no idea even IV clinics existed. Then three different people suggested I go there and do a glutathione drip, which sounded really weird and gross at first, but when three different people suggest you do something it sort of gets you thinking. (Actually, all they suggested was I do "the drip," because no one can pronounce glutathione.) I probably would have drunk my own urine at that point if three different people suggested it would fix things, which I realize would have also been really weird and gross, but at least my veins wouldn't be getting stabbed.

Here's what I know is going in: glutathione (gloo-ta-THIGH-own) is a molecule made of three amino acids—a tripeptide—and you need it. They call it "the mother of all antioxidants." Heavy metals and toxins bind to it and that's how they normally leave your body. And for whatever reason, some people don't have enough of it naturally and then you end up with a mess of problems thanks to your ever-weakening immune system. Name any illness, and whoever has it likely has a glutathione deficiency. Then you get to take your broken brain to the IV clinic where they can intravenously shoot it straight into your blood stream and everybody hopes for the best.

That being, it'll fix you. Anything to fix you. And then you will feel beautiful again.

Because Parkinson's is weird and gross.

Other thoughts:

It's not really Parkinson's. A huge mistake has been made and I might actually have grounds for a lawsuit.

Maybe this whole thing will heighten my senses, like when you go deaf or blind and everything else starts working better. Although I didn't lose a sense, but still.

I might be going crazy.

I'm not going crazy, I'm in the middle of the world's longest nightmare.

I should go to New Zealand and see a Māori healer, who are totally spiritual and who I hear can heal almost anything. (Then I remember I have a fear of flying and clearly the last thing I need is more fear to deal with.)

I should get that water that Buddhist monks have blessed because they say all that positive energy affects the structure of the water crystals.

Or maybe I should just start drinking again because I

probably wouldn't care as much about all this.

I definitely *shouldn't* start drinking again because I will end up in rehab.

But if I do end up in rehab, maybe I could do a trade with them and teach yoga there.

You know what? Things aren't that bad.

Five minutes later: everything sucks.

The IV clinic is fancy and not at all what I pictured, which was basically *M*A*S*H*. Men in fatigues would be lying on rows of uncomfortable cots, their heads wrapped in gauze, one of their legs perhaps amputated, tubes running from elevated plastic sacks into to their emaciated arms. And probably a lot of moaning and groaning.

In other words, the worst.

Thankfully, the place I've just walked into doesn't look like a war tent. It's more like a wellness spa, where you'd see people walking around in terrycloth robes and drinking cucumber water from Dixie cups. Candles are burning and pretty much everything is a variant of tangerine. My immediate impression is that a feng shui expert had been there.

Now, if you've never been to one of these places, here's what will happen: a pleasant woman will greet you. When she finds out it's your first time there, she will be very, very happy for you and commend you for choosing to do the drip thing. This will be reassuring. She will then give you paperwork to fill out, and you will have a seat in an especially plush chair to do so. Next to you on the table will be a stack of pamphlets featuring smiling, healthy people who are obviously models with no diseases, and a sign: *Ask Us About Memberships!* The whole thing will be overwhelmingly optimistic. It'll also be $150 every time you do it, so the membership might have to wait. Plus, you don't know yet if it'll even do anything. The thought of this is scarier than sitting there for thirty minutes with a needle jabbed into your arm.

Once you hand in the paperwork, you will be taken to "the back" to meet a Dr. Gordon who looks exactly like a tan Superman. He will also have a completely unidentifiable accent you will spend most of your conversation trying to figure out while he asks you what bringz you in today, and all about your zymptomz, and you will tell him everything except the part that you are a woman on a rampage to banish this shit out of your body once and for all, because that would make you look ridiculous.

He, too, will get visibly excited when he finds out it's your first time. An IV virgin! So rare! And this is when the doctor who is either from Iran or Italy or possibly

Argentina will launch into a whole thing about the benefits of glutathione, namely its ability to "prevent further oxidative damage" and "retard progression of the disease." Most of the rest will go in one ear and out the other because it'll all be very science-y and if you're anything like me you don't really understand how cells work in the first place.

Next, you and your plethora of bodily deficiencies will be taken into the "drip room." It will have low lighting and comfy lounge chairs, exactly like a cruise ship at night, except one with bags of magical glutathione and tubes and needles. You will then be told to lie down and "*relawx.*" Then you'll be left all by yourself in the drip room where you will try not to think about the fact there's probably a ton of blood sitting in the next room because people also give blood there and there's nothing weirder or grosser than blood.

And right about now it might occur to you that this might be an incredibly bad idea.

And that taking a hammer to your hand might be a better one.

I didn't really want to hurt myself. I just wanted my old body back. That, and my old sense of normalcy, which may not have been all that normal to begin with, but it was nothing like this. This was the exact opposite of normal.

This was a David Lynch movie.

A redheaded nurse in scrubs walks in. She looks like a Jane, but introduces herself as something else. Then she ties one of those long rubber things around my upper arm while I start thinking about what they actually give you in the IV drip. Is it man-made glutathione? Or other people's glutathione? And how would they even extract it from someone? I guess if they can transplant a person's eyes into you, they can do just about anything.

Anyway, it's too late to ask. The needle has already punctured my vein.

"Now, try not to fidget," she says.

I immediately want to fidget.

Instead, I close my eyes and tell myself not to think about the thingy in my arm. And also how fucking strange this whole thing is.

The fact is, it's all strange. Life is strange. I'm strange. I'm the strange chick with Parkinson's who doesn't want to tell anybody and I'm not even sure why. I hadn't even told my own family yet. And when I do, I'll probably have to fudge the timing about when I found out, because it's already been three months and I'm quite sure that's way too long to keep your loved ones out of any kind of loop. But god forbid anybody know I'm flawed. Or possibly unfixable.

Unbroken

And that may have been the scariest thought of all.

Scary, and wrong.

Sometimes, you can learn something completely mind-blowing in yoga and then totally forget about it the minute you need it the most. Or just kind of choose to forget it. *I don't need no philosophy, I need fixing.* Which isn't to say nothing ever goes wrong, because it does; or that there aren't parts of you that you just can't bring yourself to accept or maybe even detest at times (which I know is a strong word but it does apply), because I'm sure there are; or that there's no such thing as catastrophe, because there is. Oh my god, there is. And sometimes all you want to do is fix it.

But here's one thing to remember: What you come looking for, you come looking with.

It's so simple. And we want to make it into a maze. And mazes, by definition, are nothing but confusing and disorienting traps. They are designed to create frustration. And we know this, but we go for it anyway, maybe because we think it couldn't possibly be that simple to just show up and do a bunch of poses and trust it'll be enough to keep the fragments of your life magically together like a sweet little puzzle. Some days it's all you can do to get yourself to yoga in the first place, let alone fathom the power of it.

Maybe you've had a long day at work. Or you almost

just got into a car accident because you were racing to get there and not paying attention. Or you went to put leggings on earlier and *hey, look at that! You've gained weight*! Which you know shouldn't really matter, not when you're going to yoga, so then you feel stupid for caring. Or it could be a billion other things. Or absolutely nothing.

Then there are the other days. The days when your very life depends on being there. Maybe you just found out your insides are being eaten alive by cancer. Or your marriage could be falling apart, proving how unlovable you are. Or maybe some other old hurt has chosen this day to bubble to the surface, something you don't dare utter to another soul, something you may have let fester so long it's actually taken on a sinister quality, and you know you probably belong in a dark bar somewhere drowning in booze and small talk with strangers. Instead, you're the person angrily walking into yoga and slamming your mat down and not bothering to pretend that everything's not mega fucked up. And in a way, that's the best person to be. At least you're in the moment.

Toward the end of my little rampage of heck, I was sitting in class one night waiting for it to begin when I saw a girl walk in. She was young, probably early twenties, blonde and sweet-looking. She also had miniature slash marks all up and down her arms. They were scars, really. She'd been a cutter.

This was a girl with nothing to hide. Her secrets were out there, written and unerasable. And she didn't have long sleeves on or an angry stare meant to be interpreted as, *turn away bitch, and don't even think about looking at me.* She was right in the middle of the room and wearing a tank top. And if you saw her practice, you'd see someone move with all the fluidity and grace of a swan.

She and I never said one word to each other that day. But that girl is the bravest person I have ever seen.

It's a good thing yoga hasn't run out of ways to repackage the same message. Sometimes you need to hear it in a different way for it to get your attention all over again. And even though I felt pretty good afterward, I never did go back to the IV clinic. I went back to yoga, slid in among the other misfits and left the rest behind.

SUTURED #2: A BRIEF GUIDE THROUGH THE YOGA SUTRAS

BOOK TWO

PORTION ON PRACTICE

1. You're on fire now, baby. You're diving deep into the study of you. You're givin' it all up to the Vastness. You're totally doing it.

2. And those pesky obstacles? Please. We're way past those.

3. Plot twist! Here come the Five Afflictions: Ignorance, Egoism, Attachment, Aversion, and Clinging to Bodily Life.

4. Ignorance is the queen bee of all. Thanks to ignorance, the others exist. It likes to breed.

5. Ignorance is claiming knowledge of a given subject when you clearly have no idea what you're talking about.

6. Egoism is a state of mind where all you can think about is yourself.

7. Attachment happens because some stuff feels so damn good that you just want more.

8. Aversion happens because some stuff feels so damn shitty that you just want less.

9. Self-preservation drives all of the above, and since the whole point of living is stayin' alive (which is also a good Bee Gees song), they tend to get out of control.

10. Now let's talk about sending these afflictions right back where they came from. Let's harpoon the alien back into space.

11. We're talking about destroying them. For good. I know you're a peaceful being and all, but some things need destroying. And we're gonna kill 'em with kindness.

12. But you should know they're in your life in the first place, thanks to whatever went on in your last lives. And they'll carry on to your next ones. So ya might want to take care of 'em now because the One keeping score doesn't miss a damn thing.

13. See that hideous insect? That could be you in your next life.

14. And it would be your own damn fault.

15. Now if you're smart, you've figured out by now how good you are at twisting things around.

16. But you can easily avoid misery.

17. Just stop thinking (insert meaningless distraction here) will make you happy.

18. Ask yourself: Do you wanna feel good, or do you wanna feel free? (Hint: It's the second one.)

19. Here's the situation. Either something new is happening, something old is happening again, something special is happening, or something is about to happen. And that's life.

20. Stop judging it.

21. There are forces trying to tell you things to get you to the next level.

22. And sometimes bad things happen because the cosmos saw an opportunity for you to learn.

23. The cosmos is actually in cahoots with the rest of the universe to teach you stuff.

24. Reminder: that's what you're doing here on Earth to begin with. To learn how to be the best you ever.

25. And once that happens, you're pretty much done down here.

26. Now I know we've already gone over this, but you have to be relentless. We're stopping at nothing and hanging tough.

27. I've got eight things for you, yo, and they're called limbs.

28. And if you follow them, you'll basically be perfect.

29. Don't diss others. Don't diss yourself. Move your body. Breathe. Withdraw. Concentrate. Meditate. Be free.

30. Not dissing others is based on nonviolence, honesty, keeping your grubby hands to yourself, not being a jealous bitch, and having self-awareness.

31. Why do you do it? Because it's the right thing to do.

32. Stay clean. Be content, like a kitty cat. Keep a fire under your ass. Learn from yourself. Accept your fate.

33. Don't go talking yourself out of these things. They're kind of important.

34. Because life's too short to be a miserable prick.

35. Happy people repel miserable pricks.

36. And people who do yoga are not miserable pricks.

37. Here is the secret to life: Not wanting stuff. Because the second you stop wanting it, that's when it all comes to you. Or you can just pretend to not want it, like in seventh grade when you pretended you didn't want Ian Holmes to notice you in your crocheted top and your Dittos but he totally did. And *that's how it's done.*

38. Life should be effortless.

39. And when you don't try to hoard stuff, you'll understand hoarding stuff makes for some bad karma.

40. And you know how great you feel after you take a shower? That's what's happening here, but emotionally. And you'll want to stay that way. Now is not the time to go rolling around in the mud.

41. Because you're starting to see it: the Truth.

42. Look at you now, all happy!

43. You're the boss of your own body. It is the mob and you're the Tony Soprano.

44. The universe is suddenly starting to make sense to you.

45. You + the Universe = One.

46. A word now about yoga poses: They should be steady and comfortable.

47. Not unstable and torturous.

48. Keep practicing, and you'll totally be like that in real life.

49. Take an inhale. Now take an exhale. Feels good, huh?

50. Just make sure to keep it smooth and silky. And don't be fooling around with funky breathing techniques without a teacher there. You can really screw yourself up.

51. So there's breathing in, breathing out, holding the breath, and then the secret fourth door: barely breathing at all.

52. They say it feels tingly, seeing how you're basically existing on energy.

53. And that is what they call *focus*.

54. You'll forget you even have a body. That's how crazy this whole thing is.

55. Man, it feels good to be in control.

What is it that dies? A log of wood dies to become a few planks. The planks die to become a chair. The chair dies to become a piece of firewood, and the firewood dies to become ash. You give different names to the different shapes the wood takes, but the basic substance is there always. If we could always remember this, we would never worry about the loss of anything.

—SWAMI SATCHIDANANDA

SEVEN

ALIVE

You know it's not good news when the phone rings at 4:30 in the morning. It never is, especially not when it's your friend Christina calling from your mother's nursing home. Had I put a little more thought into this moment ahead of time, I may have changed my ringtone to something a little less jaunty than the *Charlie's Angels'* theme song.

I sit up in bed and look at Mauro. "What should I do?"

"You should probably answer it…."

"Or maybe *you* should answer it." Yes, he definitely should answer it. Because I'm pretty sure I know what's happening, which is exactly why I had Christina stay with my mom in the first place. She's much better at this stuff than me. I suck at talking to people who take care of the ill.

"My daughter isn't very medical." My mother said this countless times over the years to doctors, surgeons, emergency room technicians, and plenty of others who stick needles into people for a living. For some reason they always assumed I wanted to hear the grim details of her situation, but this was my mother we were talking about, and honestly, the details gave me the willies. I was much better off not knowing.

Stroke?

OK, thanks. That's all you had to say.

Advancing dementia? Weak bones? Aortic aneurysm?

La-la-la-la-la-la-la-la I can't hear you, hey mom let's go to lunch.

And yesterday. I'm brave-facing it at the nursing home, talking to the hospice guy who's telling me she's slipped into a coma, and at this point it's only a matter of hours. She's "actively dying," he says. Okay, what the hell was *that?* The scariest sounding oxymoron ever, that's what. I'd almost rather get lied to, or at least euphemism-ed. "Transitioning" would have been just fine, or even "winding down." This is when I learn what the letters DNR stand for: Do Not Resuscitate.

"I'll stay overnight," Christina offered. This is when it's good to have a friend who's sat with dying people before. "Go home, get some sleep. If anything changes, I'll let you know."

In other words, *I'll call you if she dies.*

By the time Mauro picks up the phone, I feel like it's been ringing for an hour. "Hey Christina…" he says, then yeah, she's right here, and then okay, okay, and maybe an uh-huh and then another okay, and by the time it all melts into wuwah-wuwah-wuwah it doesn't take much to figure it out from there.

Trust me when I say this will be the most warped split second of your entire life. It starts off almost normal. Then time somehow manages to stretch itself out like a rubber band, and by the time it snaps itself back into place the whole thing ends with the appalling realization that *you are now a motherless person.*

They hang up. Mauro looks me. "Are you all right?" He isn't sure what else to say. He's never been with anyone the moment they found out their mother just died. And am I? I have no idea.

"It's weird. I feel like she's watching me."

That's the other thing. Suddenly you feel watched. My mother is watching me from the Beyond, which means she probably saw me ignore the phone when it first rang and may have thought I couldn't be bothered to answer it because I was sleeping and, knowing my mom, her feelings would be incredibly hurt and how do you make up for that. *Sorry mom, but you know how much I hate the phone.*

The thing is, I do hate the phone. I wonder why.

"Anne, your mother is out of surgery."

"Anne, we're calling because we had to send your mother back to the hospital."

"Anne, it might be time for you and your brother to start thinking about hospice care."

Hospice care? No, you must mean Frisbee game. Because there is no way my brother and I aren't outside right now playing Frisbee in the middle of the street in the middle of summer and there are weird bugs everywhere

no matter how much bug spray we put on ourselves and
our mom is coming out to tell us for the third time and
final time, "C'mon inside kids, it's getting dark."

My brother John lives in Dallas. We'd just spent half the day on the phone together, wading through doctorspeak, making decisions we didn't want to make. And now I have to call him and tell him our mother died.

I had to call my brother and tell him our mother died.

All of a sudden, I feel way too grown up.

Now if you have to call someone with this kind of news, you should probably figure out exactly what you're going to say first. Write it down if you have to. Rehearse. You don't want to just blurt it out as soon as they answer— which my brother does on the very first ring.

"Hey…."

"Hey. It just happened. She's gone."

Or that. I couldn't help it. I've never done this before and it's still only four something in the morning. Luckily— if you want to call it that—he says he pretty much knew why I was calling, so at least I didn't *totally* shock the shit out of him. Then he asks me, "Are you okay?" And I say, "Yeah, I'm okay, you?" And John says he's okay, and then I say, "She's watching us, you know that, right?" And he says, "Oh yeah, she's watching us. She's spying on this whole conversation." And I say, "Spying!" And then we both start laughing, and I mean really laughing, and I'm not even really sure why, except to say we take after her.

"I know you must hate this, Mom." We were at the hospital, two years earlier. This time she had fallen and broken her leg while she was walking. Just walking.

"Well, it is what it is," she said. Then, "I'll give you a million dollars if you'll go get me a decent cup of coffee. You know how much I hate the coffee at Shady Pines."

"Where?"

"You know, the nursing home."

"It's called Sunny Hills, Mom."

"Oh, whatever," she said. And then she laughed at herself, because she knew how.

When I finally told my mother what was going on with me, it wasn't nearly as awful as I thought it would be. But it was still pretty awful.

"Well, this is very bad news," she kept saying. "Very bad news. This is bad."

Like I hadn't put her through enough in life. Now this.

"Don't worry about me, mom. I'll be all right."

"No, this is bad. This is really bad."

From then on I played it *way down*. Her memory wasn't that great anyway, so I kind of hoped she'd just forget about the whole thing. She didn't. But at least she stopped saying how bad it was.

So now what? It's barely light out. Do I stay up? Go back to sleep? Bust out some yoga? I'm thinking maybe I should take a moment to myself, ponder my own mortality. Or turn on the TV. A good *Twilight Zone* might be on.

Mauro says he's going to get donuts. "Please don't get in a car accident while you're gone," I tell him on his way out the door. "Not a good day."

He smiles. It's a weird smile. I can't tell if he's relieved or worried I haven't started screaming my head off yet. You'd think I'd want to punctuate the moment with something, anything, perhaps one long, guttural Dylan Thomas wail: *Rage, rage against the dying of the light!* But it's still *really* early, and I have neighbors. *And* I'm still trying to wrap my head around the absurdity of the fact that the day before she was here, and now, just one day later, she isn't. Think about it. Death is so fucking absurd.

My mother had dark brown hair and light gray eyes the color of nickels. She was the only person I ever knew with eyes that color. In her later years, once her hair turned gray as well, she could have easily passed for Judi Dench. Which means my mom was James Bond's boss. If she could fake a decent British accent, you'd never know the difference. She would try but it sounded way more like Zsa Zsa Gabor, especially if she had the chance to tell you she was born in *Beverly Hillzzz, Dahlink*. She never cussed, visited Europe, or got drunk. She wore cocktail rings on special occasions. Her name was Margery, which everyone always misspelled.

Just then the hospice people call wanting me to choose an outfit for her to be cremated in. Not ever having thought about this ahead of time, I say, "Her beige Juicy tracksuit and a pair of Uggs."

I hear a *tsk*.

Disapproval? Really? When we get off the phone I Google *what do people wear when they get cremated*, in case I'm way off the mark. Apparently, a lot of people wear their pajamas, which makes total sense. I guess I assumed people were naked, but that would be weird. And there's probably a law.

It's a perfect time to tell Mauro what to do with me if I die before him. But if I'm bad at sick talk, he's even worse at death talk. He thinks it's morbid and pointless. I remind him sometimes that everyone dies and that it's just good sense to figure some stuff out ahead of time, to which he usually responds by saying *he knows that*. It's clear he feels heckled by these chats so that's pretty much where they end. When it comes to it, I might just have to have a letter prepared with instructions as far as outfits and other final wishes. If he goes first, I'll probably just have to wing it.

My father was an estate planner. Warren Ellsworth Clendening, *Esq.* He did wills for a living, although I don't know how he would have felt about doing a will for his own daughter, not that I own much that anyone would haggle over except a few great hats.

One morning, he was walking up the steps of the Santa Monica Courthouse on his way to work and had a heart attack. He died before he hit the ground. That's what the autopsy guy said. He was sixty-five.

No warning. No drawn out deathbed goodbyes. No nothing.

That was twenty years ago. I remember it like it was twenty minutes ago. And it may as well be two billion ago.

"You know what? He'll always be with you now." My friend Clare and I were in the car on the way to my parent's house that day. I wasn't in the mood for hooey, but when people say things like that you nod along and say, "I know" and "Thank you for that," even though you're really thinking, "You're actually wrong, hello, they're fucking dead" and "How is that helpful?"

Answer: it's the truth. I just didn't know it yet. It had

Alive

only been half an hour.

Up until then, aside from two dogs, a cat, and a pet mouse that was unfortunately found lifeless in the mouth of one of those dogs, I had no experience with death in the family. We never really knew if Ragamuffin was responsible for the death of that mouse or if she was trying to lick it back to life, but I never saw her as a killer. She didn't seem wily enough. Rags was born a runt, the unfortunate product of our cockapoo Gypsy and the neighbor's something—no one knew—and never had much potential as far as dogs go.

"Ragamuffin just needs a little extra love," my mother would say.

"Rags is ugly, mom." She was. Ask my brother.

"Stop it. She'll hear you."

"Yes, but she won't know what I'm saying."

She was protective. (Translation: she lied.) Now, I don't know what you were told about death when you were young, but parents can get away with saying almost anything, knowing they have years until you figure out the truth, and here's a perfect example. When I was nine my mother told me little Buffy from *Family Affair* crawled into a refrigerator, closed the door on herself, and died. How or why you would do such a thing, I have no idea. My mother, the bad chooser of normal cautionary tales, didn't want to tell me Anissa Jones had really passed away from a drug overdose at eighteen years old. Cocaine. PCP. Prescription drugs. It would have been way better than the refrigerator thing, which I'm guessing would only happen if you were on drugs anyway.

By then, my grandparents had all passed away. The singular cause of their deaths, I was told, was "old age." Apparently this was code for "cancer." I put two and two together once when I found a fancy pink lighter from the fifties that belonged to my grandmother, and that's when I finally got the whole story. Smokers. All of them. I still have that lighter, even though it's never worked.

Family outings to people's graves is something you don't hear much about anymore. It must be a seventies thing. Some cemeteries have yoga, which I think is oddly cool and very peaceful sounding, assuming they don't do it at night. (*Insert Corpse Pose joke here.) And here in L.A. they show old eighties movies at Hollywood Forever. I wonder if this might be crossing a line. If it were me buried there I don't know how I'd feel if a thousand people were stomping on my grave in a mad rush to get a good seat for *Edward Scissorhands*.

So when we were young, my parents would pile my brother and me in my father's gold Ford Thunderbird on holidays and some Sundays to go visit my grandparents' graves. In fact, I feel like we did these kinds of family outings far more often than what might be considered normal. I don't remember the four of us ever once going to a movie.

Two things: The cemetery where my grandparents are buried is not sprawling. It's tiny. It's probably as big as a city block. I took Mauro there once and at first he thought it was part of the parking lot for the bank next door.

"So where is it?"

"You're looking at it," I said. "Don't you see the headstones?"

The other thing about this cemetery is that, off in a corner where you'd never expect, is Marilyn Monroe's grave. She's actually buried in an aboveground crypt in the middle of a bunch of other people, which never made much sense to me because those things hardly looked big enough for a human, let alone a casket. And every time we went on these visits to the tiny cemetery, my mother would say, "go see if Marilyn has fresh flowers on her grave," because she read Joe DiMaggio sent roses twice a week, and sure enough, they would always be there. And I would look at those roses every time and think, *death is beautiful.*

Cut to the day my father died. Now I'm thinking, *death is fucked.*

Imagine showing up at your parents' house to find your mother, a widow for one whole hour, acting like, well, a lunatic. There was no uncontrollable sobbing, no chucking of things against the wall. She was cracking jokes. She was almost giddy. Say hi to your widowed mother! Ha ha, I'm a widow now! Her reaction to my father dropping dead was that of someone being tickled. And my brother and I were looking at each other like, what in holy hell is going on here and at what point do we call the doctor. That point came sooner than later. She was in shock, he said. Also, he had a pill for that. We'll take it.

That night, after things calmed way down and all the people who brought food had come and gone, John and I were sitting on the back patio with our mom. We had no idea what to say or do. Someone wasn't there anymore, that's all we knew. We'd gone from four to three. And then, staring up at the August sky, she said this: *I feel like he's watching us.*

Franz Kafka wrote, "The meaning of life is that it ends." Which is true in a way, if a little pessimistic. But he also wrote *The Metamorphosis*, which is one of my favorite stories. In the book, Gregor Samsa, a traveling salesman, wakes up in bed one morning surprised to find he has changed into a giant insect. His body is now hard, domed, and segmented. Multiple, pitifully thin legs have sprouted from his repulsive new shape and are flailing about. His family is horrified. The traumatized maid begs to be fired. His life is now about crawling up walls, scuttling under sofas, and eating rotten food. Why? No reason. Except some say he was kind of a bastard.

There's life, there's death, and there's karma. The phenomenon of cause and effect. Good or bad, every action or thought from this and previous states of existence determines your now, and it's considered to be a law of the universe, exactly like gravity. It's also why they say if you want to know what your pasts lives were like, look at your life now. Because you earned it. Although I'm not sure what a person has to do to earn certain stuff, but I'm convinced in one of my lives, maybe even my last one, I must have bullied someone with Parkinson's disease and whoever you are, I am really, really sorry.

From Eckhart Tolle: "The Now is as it is because it cannot be otherwise. What Buddhists have always known, physicists now confirm: there are no isolated things or events. Underneath the surface appearance, all things are interconnected." So if you want to walk around acting like a dickhead, go right ahead. But pull up a chair. You'll be here a while. Be willing to spend your next ninety thousand lives working your shit out. And round and round you'll go, stuck in the miserable and perpetual cycle of birth and death known as Samsara.

Gregor Samsa. Samsara. Yup. Kafka was into Arthur Schopenhauer, the "Father of Pessimism" and one of the first Western philosophers to study and write about Buddhism and Eastern thought. He believed in the chain of causation, that things don't just spring into existence from nothing, and that we shouldn't be all that happy about being born because the whole point of life was to accumulate enough good karma to end Samsara. The world, he said, was nothing but one big penal colony, and human beings are pathetic because we just can't learn. And he kind of had a point.

The soul is here to evolve. And in Yoga philosophy, the only way to do that is to be born in a human body with all its limitations and annoying flaws. But the soul— the *atman*—is immortal. It's a fluid, indestructible body of light that can't be hurt or destroyed. It doesn't know hunger or thirst, happiness or misery. It doesn't get sick with neurological diseases or have heart attacks. You won't see it in front of a mirror judging itself for gaining weight or hear it bitching about how it's not rich. It doesn't lie or cheat or stomp its feet when life gets shitty. The atman is never born, and it never dies.

And speaking of indestructible, here's some science. In the world of physics, there's no such thing as creating or destroying energy. No substance in the universe is ever dead. All it can do is change states. So when your time in your body comes to an end, all fifty trillion of your atoms will ricochet back into the atmosphere and get recycled into other stuff. Your carbon atoms will bind with oxygen atoms to be released in the carbon dioxide of some billy goat's exhale on a farm in Mongolia. Then someone, somewhere, will be born, breathe you in, and when they die they'll breathe you out with lungs partly made from you and me both.

Fact: You are part Shakespeare. You are part Jack the Ripper. You are part dinosaur. You are part of a star that exploded way back at the beginning of time. On one level, you've already lived forever. There is no separation. These bodies our souls live in are an assemblage of recycled parts of each other, made of the same little hurricanes of flinging matter and temporarily bound together by a mysterious electromagnetic force. "So forget Jesus," wrote the physicist Lawrence M. Krauss. "The stars died so that you could be here today."

He'll always be with you. No matter which way you look at it, my friend was right. I just hoped he wasn't pissed at me.

Here's what happens after you suddenly lose a parent at thirty years old: You get a hold of yourself long enough to get through the first part. The phone calls. The funeral. The spreading of the ashes. You want to keep the pain of it all to a dull hum.

Then a bit of time will go by, and you might find you're kind of okay. And one day someone will say something totally out of the blue, and you'll be slammed with the realization that you were the worst daughter of all time.

Maybe you didn't spend enough time with them. Or you never called them for no reason. Or to go to lunch. Or maybe you did something horrible, something you never apologized for because you figured hey, why dredge up the past. Then you conveniently forgot about it.

A year had gone by since my father passed away when my friend Shane from San Francisco came to stay with me. Next to my husband, Shane may be the coolest person I know. Think if Heath Ledger and Jack Nicholson had a kid together, then mix in a little Dylan from *Beverly Hills 90210*, add some tattoos, and toss him an electric guitar. I don't even know if Shane played guitar, but he should have.

Shane was also one of the only people I knew who did yoga. *And* he went to a studio and practiced with a teacher every day who, I assumed, knew his name. I'd only been doing yoga for six months, and at the gym. No one knew the first thing about me at the gym.

One day Shane came home from yoga, looking all chill. This was the nineties. If I didn't know better I would have said he was on quaaludes.

"Look at you," I said. "You glow."

He smiled. "Yeah, we did backbends today. They open your heart."

"How do backbends open your heart."

"Think about what happens in a backbend," he said, leaning back, like he was about to walk under a limbo stick. "Your whole front body is exposed. And vulnerable."

"...And they're hard."

"Well, you know what they say..." I didn't. But I'll never forget what he said next. "If backbends are hard for you, it means you're afraid to look back into the past."

Annnd... Sad.

Right then, I went to a day, years ago, I was sitting in a restaurant with my parents. I was eighteen or nineteen, and hungover. As usual. There was a distance, one I apparently thought needed filling, and I ended up saying something especially awful—I don't remember what—and my father got up and left. And in a tearful look back at me, I saw the one thing I regret most in my life. It was the shame and disappointment of a father who wonders how he could have raised such a monster.

Or worse, a stranger.

Of all the sorrows, regret is the heaviest. I would be sorry. I would be sober. I would do yoga. I would be sweeter, softer, happy-go-luckier, better. Time would make it easier. Time does that. The cliché is true: time heals. But I know I'll probably come back as some kind of filthy insect for that one.

One parent is long gone. Now the other one is at the mortuary, which is not at all what I expected. Mortuaries are supposed to be somber and creepy. This one looks more like a Tijuana séance chamber, with its bright purple walls and its plethora of Jesus candles and rosary beads and bedazzled crucifixes that are *on sale this week! Half off!*

This is what happens when you don't plan ahead. When you randomly choose a mortuary from a list provided by the hospice people.

Alejandro the mortician sits down with us and goes over our options. We can purchase a very nice, reasonably priced urn for the cremated remains. Or infuse the ashes in a multi-colored decorative piece of "art glass." There's burial at sea, á la the Neptune Society in an underwater, enchanted garden–like graveyard. Also, some people fashion the remains into an actual diamond.

I'm riveted by this. I make a mental sticky note to Google that diamond shit later.

We decide to go with the one that looks like a large cardboard can of beans. Her ashes are going in the ocean anyway, so why get fancy.

As I'm signing the paperwork, Alejandro launches into a series of stories we have no desire to hear. One has to do with people who spread the ashes of their loved ones at the Haunted Mansion ride at Disneyland. According to his story, the Disneyland folks couldn't seem to figure out why large amounts of dust kept mysteriously collecting.

Dust? Nope. Cremated humans.

Jesus. I need a nap.

"Are you okay?" My friend Ronna is with me.

"I'm okay, Ro."

"You seem unusually calm." Meaning, *Grieve already, ya freak.*

Things were different this time. I'd made sure of that. I was the clingiest daughter you've ever seen. Sometimes I'd call my mom three times a day just to make sure she was still alive. "Hey it's me, just checkin' on ya."

"Anne, I'm not lying here in a pool of blood," she would say. God, she was funny.

Two weeks later, we rent a boat to spread her ashes in

the ocean by the summer home we had when I was a kid. Same place as my father. Thirteen of us are there to send her off, and it's late in the afternoon, right when the sun is setting when we stop the boat. And when my brother tips that cardboard container over just enough to let the first of those ashes hit the water, just for an instant, the sky lights itself on fire and bursts into the brightest, most ravishing color of red you've ever seen.

"Look, you guys!" my then-fifteen-year-old niece Caroline yells out. "She's back together with grandpa!"

And I think, *Wow, death is beautiful.*

I have my father's dog tag from when he was in the Air Force. He used to carry it on his keys, and together they would make a very distinct and tinny jingle sound, like wind chimes might if they were made of little spoons. I carried that dog tag on my keys for years, until finally I took it off for fear I'd lose it. But you couldn't tell me a part of him wasn't alive every time I heard that sound. It's my favorite sound.

Think about who you love. Tell them how you feel. And keep an open heart, because one day we'll be unbound. And "maybe," as Arthur Miller wrote, "all one can do is hope to end up with the right regrets."

It's three days after my mother passed away, and I'm in yoga.

Toward the end of class, I make my move. Lying on my back, I bend my knees, plant my feet and place my hands next to my ears. Eyes closed, I take an inhale, push away from the earth and rise up into the backbend in one fluid, ecstatic expression of openness and heart.

Then I come down and immediately start sobbing, right there under the vastness of everything.

Luminous beings are we,
not this crude matter.

—YODA

EIGHT

TRAUMATIZED

Four days after we spread my mother's ashes in the ocean, Mauro and I decided to get married in the exact same way Demi Moore and Patrick Swayze decided to get married in *Ghost*. The only difference was we were at home, not walking on a New York City street, and no one got shot thirty seconds later. Other than that, the whole thing was pretty much identical.

Mauro had been telling me for years he would marry me one day and I always said the same thing back, that I thought marriage was old fashioned and nothing but a piece of paper and that we didn't need it. And it wasn't that I didn't love him or anything, because I did. I loved that cat so much it was unbelievable. If I could invent a person, I never would have imagined someone with such a massively huge and giving heart as his. It's astonishing. It's the human organ equivalent to every Barry Manilow song ever written. And maybe I was just being cynical, or I didn't want him bossing me around, or I just needed control over *something*, I don't really know. Or maybe I just didn't want him getting stuck with me.

I changed my mind the day we were on that boat. When you walk though death with someone, things have a way of becoming suddenly and vividly clear. He was already my family.

So on that morning, while he was sitting there

drinking coffee and looking for Porsche gadgets on Ebay and not at all expecting this next thing to come out of my mouth, I said, "You know, I think we should get married."

His face turned into saucer eyes. "Are you serious?"

"Yeah. Let's get married."

"You're serious."

"I'm serious."

I made my own dress on my grandmother's sewing machine. It was black and strapless. I also didn't finish it on time and had to be sewn into it. Mauro's mother came from Australia to stay with us and it was exactly like having a mother again because she's originally from Italy, and if you know anything about Italian mothers you know they love to take care of you and make you eat because they always think you're too thin. We ordered a chocolate and vanilla cake, a slice of which is still in my freezer even though it's way too old and gross to eat. My friends put together a bouquet of purple flowers mixed with peacock feathers for me to hold. And on New Year's Day, at eight o'clock at night in a Hollywood restaurant in front of fifty cheering friends and family, I became his wife.

It's now March, two and a half months later. I'm teaching almost every day. I'm in the middle of a three hundred-hour teaching mentorship program. I'm doing so much yoga my body looks like chiseled steel. I'm writing for an online wellness site where I'm also interning as an assistant to one of the editors, *and* I'm bartending four nights a week.

I am so at the top of my game.

Then one day I completely forget about a morning class I have to teach until five minutes before it starts. Which means I got there fifteen minutes late. This has now happened twice. And I have no idea if it's because I never write stuff down, or because I'm always at the bar until the wee hours of the morning and I'm too exhausted to keep track of everything, or if maybe the evil thing inside me is slowly but surely hammering away at my ability to remember much of anything. But I do know going senile right now (or ever) would not be at all cool and that my brand new husband deserves a wife who won't be forgetting in a year's time how to tie her own shoelaces.

So I go see neurologist #4, and we have a very lively discussion about how it's going with the medication. I tell her it's going pretty okay, but it could be going better, and she says maybe we'll add this other one and see how it goes, so I go ahead and add the other one but it ends up getting chucked in the trash three days later because it gives me the most frightening nightmares a person could possibly have. She did warn me about this ahead of time, but I laughed her off because *come on, how bad can they be*.

Soul annihilating. That's how bad. I would literally rather tape my eyes open and watch *The Silence of the Lambs* over and over for a week straight than go back on that stuff. And it wasn't even helpful, but then again I only gave it three days.

Thankfully I still have the bar, where they do burlesque shows with themes like comic book villains and *The Wizard of Oz*. You haven't seen anything until you've seen a sexy flying monkey peeling off her clothes. Or a man sprayed head to toe in silver paint and made to look like the Tin Man doing an artful pole dance. And the weirdest thing about it is it barely seems weird at this point. These are my Saturday nights at work.

My worlds are starting to clash. Like a bad plaid. Not one thing makes sense next to the other. Happy wife. Sick brain. Yoga teacher. Bar creature. Sober two and a half decades. Sometimes breezy and calm. Other times worried and frazzled.

But I just keep on truckin'.

One day I wake up not knowing where I am. All I can see is white. I want to say it's a wall, but I could be wrong.

Wait—Did I just wake up?
And what feels so heavy?
Thickness.
Whiteness.
Voices.
Where am I?

Finally, my soupy head comes to. I'm in my living room, lying on my couch, the incredibly comfortable purple velvet one that may as well be double strength Ambien. People who sound Brazilian are on TV talking about some soccer game that came on after the last thing I was watching, whatever that was. And judging from the light outside, I can see it's either late afternoon or early morning, which of course puts me in a panic because I have no clue if I'm supposed to be somewhere. Or when. Or much else.

You know you've overdone it when a nap becomes more like a coma. Or maybe my brain was just conserving energy, like what happens in a rolling blackout. I may have officially overused it.

I shake the dead-ish feeling off and look at my phone. There's a text from my friend Rose, who's also the manager of the studio where I teach.

Are you going to the trauma workshop this weekend? You haven't signed up yet.

I text her back.

I haven't decided yet.

She texts me back.

I think it would be really good for you.

(Hesitation.)

I've known about my friend Mischa's "Yoga for Trauma" workshop for weeks and just couldn't get excited. Part of it is the word: *trauma*. As in *blunt force*. There aren't many words more antagonizing-sounding than that. Also, Mischa already mentioned to me that part of the workshop is going to be a guided visualization, something I can only assume will be unpleasant considering the entire focus is on trauma, and when I hear words like *visualization* and *trauma* together the first thing I think of is the dance scene in *Jacob's Ladder* where Elizabeth Pena is grinding away with a demon. Then there's the thought of getting accidentally hypnotized, which I admit I have a slight fear of ever since I saw something happen once years ago in a bar.

There was a hypnotist. He called a woman up on stage, said a few words, snapped his fingers, and she was out. Just like that, he had total control over her. Then he told her to position herself between two chairs, so that her head was on one chair and her feet were on the other, and act like a plank of wood. Which she did. And then *he stood on her*.

All the drunk people clapped. It was an impressive spectacle. Rarely do you see a grown man standing on the stomach of a petite female while she's illogically hovering in space.

That's how fragile your mind is. And why you have to be very careful about who you let inside your head. I can't imagine what kind of sludge might come gushing out if the wrong person goes banging around up there and breaks something, and I'd spent way too much time in the recent past with a soldering gun in one hand and a roll of duct tape in the other trying to make sure that didn't happen. And I seriously doubt anyone would want to stick around and help me clean up the mess if it did.

But yoga isn't always about showing up and feeling good and jumping around just to get your mind off whatever's going on. (Maybe sometimes.) That's what gyms and bars are for. It's also not a handful of Valium, even if it does have kind of the same effect, and it's not necessarily an anesthesia for hurt. In all its variations, it's the practice of letting the sludge out. And *leaving it there*. Because here's the thing about the traumas of life, and what Peter Trachtenberg wrote in *The Book of Calamities:*

Five Questions about Suffering and Its Meaning: "You yourself are property. The property of that which has injured you." He goes on to compare it to a brand. As in the scalding kind. As in the kind they put on cattle to identify ownership. It isn't just a bitter remembrance of something painful. It is bitterness. It is pain. And it's very real.

Say something bad happens. (Your house catches on fire with you in it.) Or it happens to someone right in front of you. (Their house catches on fire with them in it.) Or you hear about something bad that happened to someone you love. (Your best friend's house catches on fire with them in it.) Or you've been repeatedly exposed to bad stuff happening. (You work in an ER where people come in all the time after getting caught in house fires.) These are the moments that create the brand. And now when you see/hear/smell fire, you'll go straight to the fear that you or someone else will burn to death—which, by the way, is a pretty legitimate fear—because you're basically reliving the whole thing. Your nervous responses can't differentiate between the then and the now. Ask any combat vet how they feel about the sound of popcorn popping in the microwave. Or the adult child of an alcoholic whose husband comes home drunk, again. And there's no use trying to talk yourself down from those moments, because no one's listening. The reptilian brain has taken over, which is the part that's all about visceral experience. And that, I ended up finding out, was the point of the visualization, to acknowledge and connect with sensory memories the brain has no language for, and to do it in a safe, nonterrifying place where the is no fire and there are no dancing demons.

One thing's for sure, everyone has something. Not everyone has a giant scar or a missing limb to show for it, but it's there. The indelible mark of *that thing*. It's that thing that will not just go away quietly. That thing you resent because it can't let one day go by without making you think about it no matter how hard you try, until you end up depressed/angry/drunk/isolated (at best), disassociated (middle), or utterly self-destructive (at worst). It's that thing that went ahead and branded you without your permission.

I'll give you one guess what my thing is. Hint: It starts with a P. And it ends with *leave me alone already, ya fuck face of a disease.*

So over it.

I finally text Rose back.

You're probably right I should go.

And Rose texts me back with a smiley face.

It's now Saturday morning. My alarm is going off. Wind chimes.

Today is workshop day.

I peel myself out of bed, leaving an empty quadrant. Three other beautiful beings are still semi-sleeping. One husband, two dogs. My little tribe.

God dammit, I love them.

I get to the studio, walk in the door and immediately feel swallowed. This is a room that could fit a small kingdom. A kingdom of thirty, to be exact.

Thirty people.

Thirty stories in search of a happy ending.

Mischa is there, of course looking calm. Mischa *is* calm. She is the exact person who should be teaching yoga for trauma, or maybe first grade. To know her is to feel hugged.

I haven't told Mischa how I'm feeling. In fact, I told her I was up for this workshop, which was a total lie. I never tell people how I'm feeling. I don't even know how I'm feeling half the time. One minute I'm having a yoga breakthrough and feeling all lotus-blossomy, and the next I'm at work and someone's yelling at me about their bar tab while a half-naked Glinda the Good Witch is doing a sultry dance to a punk remix of "Somewhere over the Rainbow."

I'm looking into places with sensory deprivation tanks. I think it might help.

Once we're all lined up at the wall, we start with some gentle yoga. It's nice. I never do gentle yoga. For a minute there I start judging myself for never doing gentle yoga until I remind myself that is not the point of yoga for trauma. And after twenty minutes of nice yoga, Mischa tells us to lie down and get comfortable with our feet touching the wall for the visualization. The idea is touching the wall provides sensory information through your feet so you feel "embodied," as opposed to just floating there, which is also nice. I definitely don't want to just float there.

"Now close your eyes," she says. "And envision a beautiful place, real or imaginary."

The first thing I see is an island. This is the island with the bay where we spread my parents' ashes, the one where I spent my summers growing up, and on this island there is a certain corner. And it is mine. It is the one thing on Earth that is wholly and completely mine. I laid claim to it when I was five. And on this corner, where you can sit on the seawall and let your legs dangle so your feet will *just* hit the water if it's high tide, you can see everything that could ever be worth seeing—the boats anchored out in the bay, the twinkling of sunlight when it hits the water, a Ferris wheel in the distance. Sometimes I can't believe it is real. Everything about it is beautiful.

"Now, notice the air…" Mischa says.

The air feels crisp and salty, the way sea air does.

"And the smell of it…"

Moss. The island smells of moss. And bait.

"And the sounds…"

I hear the clanking of masts, the water lapping up on the sand.

"And the light…"

It's dusk. My favorite time of day.

And this is when something amazing happens.

Mischa tells us to imagine a benevolent being, someone who knows you and who supports you. And right then my parents show up. They're sitting there with me, on my corner, the one I love so much and I was born to sit on. And I was born because of them.

"And imagine now, this being has something to tell you…"

I don't know which one said it. Probably both. Definitely both. And this is what they said:

"This is all for you…"

Over and over.

"This is all for you…"

"This is all for you…"

It was my island. My water, my sand, everything. Almost as if they had created it for me and me alone, and no one else could even see it. And because it was my vision, I knew they were also talking about everything else in my life I loved, because even though it all felt like such chaos sometimes and completely lacking sense, the truth was the good parts outweighed the rest by probably a billion. Or more. Which is why I started crying right there in Yoga for Trauma and not even caring what the two people next to me thought. Hopefully they were on their own island. And hopefully they weren't alone.

The mind is such a mystery. You could be Albert Einstein and still not fully understand the way it works. And maybe we should all be okay with that, since Einstein's the one who said, "The most beautiful thing we can experience is the mysterious." And that beauty's all for you.

Why do you go away? So that you can come back. So that you can see the place you came from with new eyes and extra colors. And the people there see you differently, too. Coming back to where you started is not the same as never leaving.

—TERRY PRATCHETT,

A Hat Full of Sky

NINE

FAR
AWAY

It's a rainy April morning, one month later, and I'm standing in front of a rental car place in San Francisco with Mauro trying to not sob.

"I don't want to go," I tell him. I may have even stomped my foot.

"Come on, you'll do great. And it's only five days."

"I don't want to go."

(sniffle.)

No, I'm not going off to jail. I'm going to a qigong retreat in Northern California. And he's driving home to L.A. Lucky bastard.

The whole retreat thing came about a few months earlier after I read an article about a woman named Rebecca who said she used to have Parkinson's and didn't anymore. She said she had taken up a practice called zhineng qigong and totally got rid of it. She wasn't on medication anymore or anything. Rebecca had baffled science.

Rebecca was obviously full of shit.

I've attempted everything I could think of to kill this thing off and nothing worked. I am a failed assassin. The only thing that's come close is yoga, because yoga calms your nervous system down and that's half the battle, but in the end it's like an annoying ant infestation that you can never really get rid of no matter how many coffee grounds you throw around or how much Raid you use. Except it's not in your kitchen. It's under your skin.

But after poking around on Rebecca's blog, I started to get the feeling she wasn't a psychopath. She seemed pretty genuine. And she looked a like an older Grace Slick, who I love. So one day I bit the bullet and sent her a very nice email demanding to know everything.

An hour later Rebecca got back to me with the most extensive email I've ever gotten from a stranger. Information and links galore. And this is what I learned:

Zhineng qigong (literal translation: cultivating intelligent energy ability), also called Chinese yoga, is a healing discipline that uses breath awareness, movement, sound, and conscious intention to clear energy blockages that cause imbalance and ultimately make you sick. In China they call it "qigong for incurables." The idea is to consciously access the "inner medicine" inside you capable of curing almost any chronic or complicated disease, to increase awareness of the relationship between you and the natural world, and to learn to guide qi (or chi, which yoga calls prana), the energy inside you that differentiates life from death. All of this, based on Hunyuan Entirety Theory.

According to Hunyuan Entirety Theory, everything in the universe, whether it's matter (the physical), or something invisible (like heat or light) can be effected or even transformed by hunyuan chi. This is the primordial energy we think of as consciousness, the highest form being human consciousness. So your mind influences your body. Energy can turn to matter, and vice versa. But hunyuan chi is the one thing that remains constant.

Qigong itself is the foundation of martial arts. And just like yoga and meditation, it increases the abundance and complexity of connections in the microstructure of white matter in the part of the brain responsible for coordination between your muscles and your limbs. So even if you aren't necessarily stronger than the next person, your body's working better, which is exactly why Bruce Lee could demolish a plank of wood by punching it from an inch away. It was less about physical strength, and more about energy. And that's the energy that had healed Rebecca.

Not seeing a reason to wait one minute, I immediately signed up for a qigong retreat. Five days and four nights in the middle of nowhere, being all healthy, kickin' it in my own redwood cabin with a fireplace and a deck where I'd drink tea in the mornings gazing at a contemplative lake. Maybe they'd have mud baths and natural spring spas and peacocks strutting around. My entertainment would be falling leaves. I'd go to bed before four in the morning.

Except now I don't want to. Somehow I totally forgot

that I hate retreats.

I like pavement. I like noise and overwhelmingly tall structures and honking taxis. I want to go to a greasy diner and get charged $5.50 for a bad cup of decaf by a disgruntled waitress. And right now all I want to do is stay in San Francisco where Mauro and I have been running for three days and finish the thing we were calling our honeymoon.

"Let's stay. C'mon, we'll go to Haight Ashbury and eat crepes."

He takes my face. "I'll call you when I get home."

It is now drizzling. It's like a poem.

In an attempt to fuse our molecules together, I hug my husband way too long. I believe this is the saddest any person has ever been in San Francisco.

"You're gonna do great," he repeats.

"I know."

(sniffle.)

Day One

I roll in late to the retreat place. It is not fancy. I will later tell people it reminds me of the compound in Waco where David Koresh and the Branch Davidians were massacred, except much smaller and with a little more greenery. I see no redwood cabins, no exotic animals.

And now I'm wondering what I've gotten myself into.

For a second I consider acting like I'm lost. There's a guy standing there looking helpful. I could ask him how to get back to the freeway and then totally bail, assuming they'd give me my money back, which is unlikely, so instead I park the car and hurriedly make my way across the gravel lot toward what I think is the entrance to the big fat ugly building. Clearly it is. Two women are standing there, looking eager.

"Welcome!"

"Hi there!"

Immediately I wonder what diseases they might have. Chronic fatigue? MS? Lyme? They look awfully healthy.

I tell the greeters how sorry I am for being late. You don't want to get off on the wrong foot by having people thinking you're the rude city chick who doesn't give a shit about being on time, unlike the forty other people I can see sitting in the room right there next to them. Fifteen minutes in, and I'm already failing.

"Oh, don't worry about it, honey."

I turn and look at the greeter who just said this, and I notice it. She's the spitting image of my mother. I can't believe I didn't see it already. She has the same face, same coloring, everything. She's even the same height. Plus, she called me honey. My mom called everyone honey.

Both of my parents are gone, but I see them everywhere. And usually when I least expect it. Sometimes it's in the subtle quirk of someone's personality, a certain lilt in their voice, or the way they walk, or if they take their coffee black because they both liked their coffee black. And it automatically makes me love them. I actually used to have a soft spot for Dick Cheney because he looked exactly like my father.

For a second I think about throwing my arms around the woman, but it's a little early on and inappropriate for that kind of thing. I decide instead to venture into the humongous room, where all the people are listening to the qigong master talk, and plant myself in a seat as non-disruptively as I can. The fact that the chairs are the loud metal folding kind doesn't make this easy, but no one really seems to care. I think they're just glad they're not the ones who were late.

Now sandwiched, I try to catch up with the action. Master Zhou, who is from China and has a very deep voice, is speaking about intention.

"If you're here thinking this won't work for you, then it won't," he's saying. "You might come with stress, you come wanting something to be different, you come maybe not appreciating what you have already. But we're here to find out what you *can* do with what you have."

I don't know what I think. I'm still not even sure what I've gotten myself into. Half of me is still standing in the rain with Mauro. Half of the other half is back at home. Half of half of half is wishing I didn't have to be there in the first place. And the last part is kind of there, but not really, and what I do know is that bringing an eighth of me probably won't suffice, not when you're on a retreat where the entire point is to manifest ridiculous amounts of healing energy to help you get over your incurable illness. But I'd never half assed anything in my life, except maybe the SATs, and that only because I was convinced they didn't matter that much. And now was not the time to start.

At least everyone else looks equally as uncomfortable. This includes the man next to me, a large man with suspenders on, who, it ends up, has had MS for ten years. I know this because right then we're told to turn to the person next to us and let them know why we we're there. I whisper back to him: *I have Parkinson's*. Then I spend the next half an hour alternately wondering if I'd rather have Parkinson's or MS and whether or not my dogs miss me. All the while Master Zhao is talking about intention and how important it is.

Okay then. My intention: stay.

The rest of the day is spent remaining positive about our diseases and getting into the practice, which is half like Kundalini and half like *kung fu* in slo-mo. And we chant, which is kind of awesome because you get to lie down and close your eyes when you do it. By the time we're done for the night, I'm worn out and it's only 9:30.

If I were home, I'd just be getting to work at the bar. But I'm six hundred miles away and I'm pretty sure I have an ear infection. I crawl into bed and Google nearby hospitals.

Day Two

I wake up at 6:40 a.m. and do twenty minutes of yoga. I don't think I've ever done yoga that early in the morning, but I'm far away on a retreat where there's absolutely no sense of time. It may as well be noon. Then I make my way downstairs to the kitchen where I'm surprised to see coffee on. *Thank the lordy.* I didn't think they'd have it. I pour myself a cup of half coffee and half water.

We do our morning practice. It ends in a dance off.

So if day one was awkward, day two is knowing you are now committed to the awkwardness and there's no turning back. I spend my time reminding myself that it's a much less awkward situation than feeling like your insides are being attacked by an invisible throng of velociraptors and that I should just go with it.

All day long we listen to more lectures on intention. I'm beginning to sense a theme. It's almost as if *he knows how easy it is to forget.* I've been to many a yoga class where I was asked to set an intention in the beginning and have never gone back to it. So now that it's a new day, I've decided to change it: get well. Not get perfect or anything, because perfect is something that flew out the window a while ago, just well. Or well-ish. Good enough.

I've also started talking to people. Ends up, most of them have MS. And most of those people are from Northern California, which could either mean they're part of an unfortunate cluster or people everywhere have MS and I never realized it. No one else there has Parkinson's. Not only have I been studying people for signs, but the woman who looks like my mother told me one day no one else had Parkinson's. I wonder if they miss their families as much as I do.

At one point we're given a piece of paper and asked to write down the things in our lives we can't seem to accept.

My list:

I'm getting older.

That's it.

Getting older really bugs me. They say age is only in your mind, but really, it's on your driver's license. Thanks to yoga I can accept almost anything, including the fact that I'm dealing with the unbelievable bullshit that's going on with me, but I draw the line when it comes to getting older. Because older means weaker. And weaker means sicker. And sicker means closer to death.

J. M. Barrie wrote the line, "The life of every man is a diary in which he means to write one story, and writes another." Clearly I never meant for this to happen, but I did know I wasn't ready for it to be over. If anything, I wanted to stop for a minute and think. Which I guess is what retreats are for.

That night we do a Yoga nidra meditation with Master Zhou. Also called yogic sleep, Yoga Nidra is that state of consciousness between waking and sleeping, where your body is totally relaxed while your mind remains awake. It's like tricking your body into thinking it's been tranquilized. What also helps is Master Zhou's voice has now somehow gotten even deeper and more commanding, like a soothing Darth Vader.

"Feeling your body as your home, relaxing from the

inside out, from the formed to the formless...."

Not one part of me is moving. I'm starting to feel encouraged.

Day Three

I get up at 6:00 a.m., do some yoga, and I'm downstairs by 6:45 for practice where we work on envisioning a healthy body with Master Zhou. Afterward the woman who looks like my mother asks me if I want to have a session with the body healer who's coming. Even though I have no idea what this entails, I say yes. And since the body healer only takes cash, that means I have to leave and go find an ATM.

It's been exactly forty-eight hours since I got there. And now I'm on a country road, passing cows, on my way back to the real world. It's odd. This should have been my chance to bust out of there and head home, but I don't feel like it anymore. I got used to being away awfully fast.

I find a gas station, use the ATM, buy myself a mini pecan pie, and go back.

Later I go to a spa-type room to meet the body healer. She looks exactly like a body healer. She has long gray hair and kind eyes. I want to tell her everything.

Once she finds out why I'm there, she has me lie back on a massage table and close my eyes. Then she starts talking to me about my kidneys. Or more specifically, about my apparent lack of kidney energy, which has led to my problem in the first place.

In Chinese medicine, *yin* essence is fluid. It's the dark side of the yin/yang symbol, the passive, softer side. It nourishes the organs and cools the body. When yin is depleted, usually thanks to stress—also, excessive fear— your body starts to heat up and dry out. And since kidney yin is the primary source of the body's yin substances, your kidneys end up drained. Then everything starts to malfunction, including your liver, which is supposed to be regulating your blood supply, and not having enough blood means the tissues in your brain become undernourished to the point where they actually start degenerating and this is when the system really breaks down. Qi is now moving so erratically through your poor whacked-out body that the phenomenon called wind happens and that is a perfect way to end up with Parkinson's disease.

Next she tells me to envision an ocean. An expansive, deep blue ocean, the bluest blue I can possibly imagine. And I'm to see this ocean inside my system, washing through me, energy as liquid blue light flowing everywhere, tumbling its way down every vein and flooding every organ with the blueness of it.

I loosen. And the moment that happens, the body worker tells me she can see thousands of lotus flowers bursting open inside me.

I leave with the most hope I've had since this whole thing began.

At 6:00 p.m. that night, we go into Noble Silence. No talking for twenty-four hours. This makes for a slightly awkward dinner with everyone, but at least there's no pressure to make small talk. Later I Skype Mauro and we have a very one-sided conversation because he's the only one who can say anything. We both think it would be funny if I start screaming at the top of my lungs, but I don't.

Day Four

I have achieved the unique ability to guess who will break Noble Silence before they open their mouth.

I, however, have remained quiet, partly because it's a challenge, and partly because I feel like I'm going to get in trouble if I don't. This is easily the longest I've ever been without speech in my entire life. It's kind of a relief. I might have to start doing this like, once a week.

So with no one to talk to, I've been walking outside for the first time since I've been here. I'm on a retreat, and that's what you do on retreats. You should go walking outside. I've also been sitting in the little library reading a qigong book, one I still have, and in it is a quote from Bruce Lipton who wrote *The Biology of Belief*: "Genes/DNA do not control our biology. DNA is controlled by extracellular signals, including the energetic messages emanating from our positive and negative thoughts. By retraining our minds to create healthy beliefs, we can change the physiology of our trillion-celled bodies."

I know how Rebecca did it. She did it by believing in it and not acting like a whiny little brat when presented with something none of us may understand. But obviously this has something to it if it's worked for so many others, and that should be proof enough for anyone. I don't really understand how electricity works, but I don't question it when I turn on a lamp. And I'll never understand quantum physics. I have no idea what Schrödinger was trying to say about that damn cat. I know he wanted to put it in a box with a vial of poison and some kind of radioactive thing so we could all be sitting around eighty years later contemplating if it's really dead or not if you can't see its blown-up lifeless body assuming the thing even went off, and that two or more realities could be occurring at once, you *just don't know*, but jesus, dude.

The reality is it happens all the time. People cure their own rare forms of cancer and run marathons after being told they'll never walk again thanks to a spinal cord injury. They shrink their malignant tumors with their mind. They go into spontaneous remission from AIDS and walk away from plane crashes. I read about a man once who got struck by lightning *seven times*. Now he's in the *Guinness Book of Records* for it. Others come to yoga, their nervous systems completely shot from anxiety or depression or some horrible illness, and the next thing you know they're flying through sun salutations. And they definitely didn't do it by sitting around acting like negative nellies.

I'm still here. Yoga is here. Intention is here. The truth is here. We're still silent.

Noble silence ends at dinnertime. I pack my bags afterward. Mixed emotions. Can't sleep.

That night I have a dream. I've been here before. I knew my teachers. One by one they appear in the dream, where we're in that big fat ugly building having tea or doing our practice or whatever, and we're not in the past but in the now, and if there's any truth to alternate realities that dream may have been all the proof I needed. And no cats died.

The next morning I tell this story to the woman who looks like my mother. She is not at all surprised. "Oh we go way, way back, honey. Lifetimes. We're connected, all right."

Day Five

I wake up at 6:30 and get myself downstairs at 7:00 for the last practice of the retreat. I'm supposed to be on the road in an hour, which I am not, because it takes me way too long to say goodbye to everyone. I want them all to caravan back to L.A. with me. By the time I finally walk out of there I'm a silly, crying mess. Twenty minutes later, I'm still a mess, and on my way home.

It's sundown by the time I make it. I dump my bags down right inside the door and do that thing you do when you've been gone from home too long, which is hug my husband and my dogs hard enough to suffocate them and stare at everything for an hour and think about how grateful I am to see it all again. It's only been a week, but I feel like I've been gone for a year.

Then I crawl into bed, set my alarm for 6:45, and crash.

SUTURED #3: A BRIEF GUIDE THROUGH THE YOGA SUTRAS

BOOK THREE

PORTION ON ACCOMPLISHMENTS

1. Start by staring at something. Anything. A random flower. A Pepsi can. A cupcake. This is called Concentration.

2. Do this long enough, and you will totally forget where you are, let alone the fact that time and space exist. This is called Meditation.

3. The most intense version of this is when you feel like you and that thing have basically warped into each other and become one thing.

4. The above three things go together, because good things always come in threes.

5. Now you have insight into that thing you were staring at. You have unearthed an ancient secret. You're Indiana Jones.

6. You have to go in order though. Seriously, start with the cupcake.

7. Remember all the stuff we did before this? Like when we were talking about you not being your thoughts? That was nothing. This stuff is way deeper.

8. And it gets even deeeeeeper....

9. And then, right when you think you've dropped all your old sucky habits, new sucky habits will swoop in and replace them.

10. But you'll get over them pretty fast, because you've been practicing your head off.

11. But ya gotta keep going. Fall down seven times, get up eight.

12. And look at both sides of the situation. There's a good side and a bad side to everything. A sweet side and a salty one. A yin and a yang.

13. The way you deal with the last three things is the way you deal with everything.

14. And let this blow your mind: before a moment happens, it's hovering in a state of "about to happen."

15. And time is the universe's way of keeping everything from happening at once.

16. Once you wrap your head around that, you'll totally see time differently.

17. And the nature of words. Because words are really just sound vibrations that kind of make no sense on their own, but we all use them.

18. Then there's reincarnation, aka Hey you! Welcome back!

19. And by understanding yourself, you'll understand other people better. It's called empathy. Unless you're a psychopath, in which case skip this one.

20. Unfortunately though, you'll never really know what others are thinking. Nor they you. You're safe.

21. You can, however, manipulate people's minds into not seeing you. (Told ya. Deeeeper....) We're talking some real JEDI SHIT here. Hypnotists do it all the time.

22. Same goes for them touching, tasting, or smelling you.

23. Now for Karma. Karma can be fast or slow, but if you're really paying attention to how you're acting, you'll start to see signs telling you how you're going to die.

24. But that's okay, you're stayin' super chill Daddy-O— which, reminder, is the whole point of all this.

25. And shit's gonna keep on happening, so you might want to go sit at the zoo and meditate on an elephant. 'Cuz they're pretty darn strong.

26. Or even something far away....

27. Think of the sun, that big burning orange thing in the morning sky, and flashes of insight will come to you about the Earth.

28. Think of the moon, that cool blue thing in the evening sky, and flashes of insight will come to you about the stars.

29. Think of the north star, which basically stays in the same

place in the sky, and flashes of insight will come to you about motion.

30. Think of the solar plexus, right in the middle of you, and flashes of insight will come to you about the structure and organization of the human body.

31. Think of that soft spot at the pit of your throat and you won't be hungry or thirsty.

32. Think of your thyroid, and you will know stillness.

33. Think of a light on the top of your head, and the knowledge of the masters will infuse your brain.

34. When all these happen at once, you'll be all, Woah.

35. Oh, and one last one: think of the heart, the thing pumping away right now inside you, and flashes of insight will come to you about the mind.

36. Question: Wanna know what makes something exist?

37. Answer: if you can hear it, touch it, see it, taste it, smell it, and/or you just have a hunch, then it probably does exist.

38. Dude, that was an obstacle. And now you just tripped yourself up. It was the obstacle of identifying things in a limited way. Focus!

39. Now look deep into my eyes. Because we, you and me, now have the ability to become each other. And we're not even on drugs.

40. When feeling heavy, take a deep breath in. Then let it out. You'll be much lighter.

41. And if you concentrate your energy on your belly button, that energy will radiate out to all the other areas because it's basically in the middle of you.

42. You're so in tune with your body by now, you're even starting to hear better.

43. And sometimes, on a good day, you might even feel like you're flying.

44. Because now you know you are so not this thing we call the body.

45. You also know that things aren't what they appear. Like that bunch of atoms over there, aka that table.

46. Right about now it will occur to you: I am indestructible.

47. And you are. You're also beautiful, and graceful, and strong, and infinitely unbreakable.

48. You're also starting to understand what's up with your insides. As in your organs. Take care of them, that's your family in there.

49. Did you know yoga would be this intense?

50. Think of a pencil, and know this: a pencil is only a pencil because your consciousness is telling you it's a pencil.

51. It's a process of undoing.

52. You've come a long way, baby. But don't get all cocky, 'cuz that's just going backward.

53. And speaking of which, time is so bizarre.

54. Think about it: Every single moment that ever happens is completely unique. And no moment that has ever happened can ever be repeated.

55. Once you see it like that, you transcend it.

56. And Ultimate Liberation will be yours. Capital U. Capital L.

nodus tollens: n. the realization that the plot of your life doesn't make sense to you anymore—that although you thought you were following the arc of the story, you keep finding yourself immersed in passages you don't understand, that don't even seem to belong in the same genre—which requires you to go back and reread the chapters you had originally skimmed to get to the good parts, only to learn that all along you were supposed to choose your own adventure.

—JOHN KOENIG,
The Dictionary of Obscure Sorrows

TEN

UNCHANGED

"So, Anne, how would you describe the tremor?"

I'm perched on yet another bed/slab thing discussing my symptoms with a neurologist who's easily ten years younger than me. *This guy has actually touched people's brains,* I'm thinking. Two other doctors flank him, creating a semicircle of white coats. Both are petite females; both remain quiet as they take notes and stare. I have the feeling I'm research.

"I'd say the tremor was incredibly annoying."

"OK, annoying *how,* exactly?" Apparently I'm not being specific enough.

"It never really goes away."

"Is there a difference when you're moving around, as opposed to sitting still?"

"Not really."

He nods. They always nod. Like they know what I mean. "And are daily tasks becoming difficult?"

I hate questions like this. There's subtext. I feel like he's implying my motor skills are about to hit the skids and before I know it I'll be one of those people who won't be able to manage opening a can of 7-Up. And then I'll have no choice but to hand it to someone to open it for me, assuming there will be anyone left in my life who still comes around from time to time to check on me, except for maybe a paid nurse who may or may not be there, and I will look at them all frustrated with my E.T. eyes as if to say, *Will you help me open this? Because daily tasks have become difficult.*

"No," I say, probably a little too emphatically. "I wouldn't say they're difficult."

Another assistant walks in. They come and go a lot. It's a nice distraction away from all the tremor talk. I see the embroidered name on her coat says Annie and I wonder how inappropriate it would be for me to offer her money for it. A little souvenir from my day of fun at UCLA medical center.

Neurologist #5 is a childhood friend of my friend Natalie. "Have you ever thought about having brain surgery?" she asked me one day. "Because I know someone who does it."

I had *not* thought about having brain surgery. Ever. And it sounded like a pretty drastic option. But she also said this guy was supposed to be the best, so I figured it couldn't hurt to just go see him and find out what he had to say, because how often are you in a position where you might need brain surgery and someone offers you a hook up out of the blue.

It may have been over the minute I got to the neurology center and saw that it was called the "neurology center." This is a structure that exists for the sole purpose of prodding around people's broken brains. It's also the most sterile environment I've ever seen. And excessively bright. The white walls, the obnoxious lighting, the shellacked flooring, everything. It could double as an interrogation space for suspected spies. I did see a vase with an orange orchid in the reception area on my way in, obviously someone's attempt to add a splash of color amidst the barrenness. But I think it was plastic.

"OK, Anne," the doctor continues. "Any problems on your medication?"

"No."

"Any hallucinations?"

"No." That's the other thing they always ask. Can't wait 'til those start.

"Any difficulty sleeping?"

"No."

"And would you say you were depressed?"

"No."

"No...?"

Rewind. "Well," I drop my chin, just slightly. "Maybe sometimes...."

I'm not depressed. I just want this shit to stop. Unfortunately you can't just march in to UCLA medical center and demand they do brain surgery on you. They actually have to *approve* you first, and something tells me they won't be doing that if I don't start acting a little more desperate.

Considering the situation, this shouldn't have been that big of a stretch. I should have been beside myself. I should have been doing laps around that whole neurology center screaming at the top of my lungs and knocking over the fake plants and maybe even flinging feces at people until they were forced to call campus security and have me hauled out of there. Then maybe I'd go visit my high school, which was *across the street*, and given everyone there a mouthful about what they had to look forward to in life.

Your education will not save you. It won't mean squat if you get sick, and you will get sick, you guys. This will lead to an existential crisis of monumental proportions, at which point you will feel alternately terror stricken, disillusioned, unlovable, disheartened, lonely, and besieged with vexing thoughts of despair coupled with sorrow. If I were you I would start stocking up on antidepressants. Now. Because you're gonna need 'em.

Oddly enough, I wasn't feeling that way. I rarely am anymore, at least not to that extreme. The wrecking ball had to stop swinging out of control at some point, and maybe I'd weighted it down with enough yoga that it finally started to slow down all on its own. The facts of the matter definitely hadn't changed. But something else had, or maybe everything was on its way to going back to being what it was before this whole nightmare started, back when I had a normal and not-so-insane amount of malcontent. And who's to say how much of it I brought on myself. Probably most. Nobody else seemed to be punishing me but me.

In Samuel Butler's novel *Erewhon*, sick people actually *are* punished. It's about a twisted, wanna be utopian society in the far realms of England where you have to sign a document at birth acknowledging you were born of your own free will and that you alone are responsible for any kind of sickness you might come down with. Also, your parents reserve the right to kill you any time they want. Robbers and murderers are taken to hospitals to "recover" while the ill are tried and thrown in prison for being morally corrupt. Even sadness counts, because grief is a sign of misfortune, and everyone is considered punishable for the actions that made them unfortunate in the first place. Hence the document.

As dark and ridiculous as it sounds, there's truth there. We put ourselves in our own little pop-up prisons. One might be for a broken heart, one for regret, one for disappointment, one for anger, one for loneliness, one for when everything is simply fucking putrid, and maybe even one for when you just don't feel at all like dealing. It does hurt to know you're responsible for your own messes, even if you aren't necessarily the one who started them. Sometimes it all makes no sense whatsoever, and at the same time there's nothing less sensible than beating yourself up when you're down.

The philosopher Lao Tzu said, "Life is a series of natural and spontaneous changes. Don't resist them; that only creates sorrow. Let reality be reality. Let things flow naturally forward in whatever way they like." You really don't have much choice anyway. Maybe in my *Fantasy Island* version of life, where everything is super easy and fun and beautiful every single minute and nothing ever goes wrong. There's also no such thing as pain of any kind, no illness, no self-doubt. I am not affected by adversity because it doesn't exist. I also don't ever age, say the wrong thing, gain weight, have anxiety, or make stupid mistakes. I am untouchable. I am a total fucking Jedi.

And then there's the flip side: reality.

At first I was totally up for brain surgery. Why not. People have it all the time, and chances were I'd come out fine. Although I did get a little weird when I found out what it entailed.

"It's called deep brain stimulation," one of the doctors explained. This sounded vaguely sexual to me, but it's not. It's where they open up your skull, stick a bunch of electrodes on your brain and then attach them to a battery-operated thingy that sits under your collar bone and sends electrical impulses all up in there. Then, *bam!* There goes 80 percent of your Parkinson's symptoms.

Another one chimed in with even better news. "And you're awake the whole time."

Yikes. "You're awake?"

Yes, you're awake. I saw a YouTube video of it once. A guy had the same surgery done, while he was playing guitar. This is so they can make sure they put everything in the right place inside your body and that it's all working. You definitely don't want them to close you up and have it end up being wrong.

So I start picturing it: First, they'll have to shave my head. Or worse, just a part of it, which I'll have no choice but to play off as a cool eighties thing. Dale Bozzio from Missing Persons did it and it was rad. Then they'll clamp my head into some contraption and Medusa me up to a million wires, at which point they'll have my husband sign the necessary paperwork "in case of anything" and he'll collapse in a heap, saying "I can't do this" and everyone will be rubbing his arm telling him it's going to be fine. Then he'll pace up and down in the waiting room while my friends watch the whole thing from a glassed off observation room. And wave at me. And take video. I actually ran this by them and they agreed that's pretty much what they would do. Then there's my friend Jalee, who is a psychotherapist and in love with brains, who told me if I went through with this, she would want to be in the room during the surgery. I told her that would be fine and that she could touch my brain if she was very, very careful.

"So, Anne. Do you have any questions for us?" Neurologist #5 and his two sidekicks are all staring at me. It's like they want to get started. Right now.

I tell the doctor I need to think about it and that I have to split. I have a class to teach in less than half an hour, and the studio is half an hour away, so now I have to double time it because there's no way I can be late to teach. And I don't know what I'd even say. *Sorry, guys. I was at UCLA talking to the neurologist about brain surgery.*

I wonder if they'd even believe me. I suppose I could have pulled a good class theme out of the situation, maybe something about going with the flow or not hating life when things get fucked up, both of which I think sum up the whole point of yoga pretty darn well, even if one is a tad less poetic than the other. Sometimes, though, you just don't feel like a poet.

I leave with a head full of brain talk and a stomachache. And seven minutes later I'm careening down Sunset, playing beat the clock, thinking about everything that's happened and everything that's changed, which is too much, when it occurs to me what *hasn't* changed, because—and this is something, in a different sense, I can't say very often—I know exactly where I am. I'm on a road I've driven a million and a half times. I know every twist and turn of it. It's been that way ever since I was sixteen years old joyriding in my brother's Cougar. I could probably drive it blindfolded and still get to the studio okay. And I'm sure if I were anywhere else in that moment, somewhere unfamiliar, I may have let myself get all overwhelmed with loneliness and lostness like you do when too much changes at once, but getting lost is what happens to stuff around the house and I am not a mislaid pen. I'm right there, and that'll never change.

I get to the studio with a minute to spare. I've almost forgotten about the whole thing. (*Almost.*) I start class with a few words about gratitude, and from there we flow.

And now how do I feel about brain surgery?

Sigh.

I don't know. I'm still on the fence.

Sometimes people let the same problem
make them miserable for years
when they could just say, *So what.*
That's one of my favorite things to say. *So what.*

— ANDY WARHOL

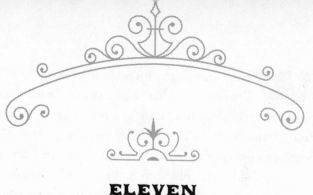

ELEVEN

HAPPY

When I was young I wanted to grow up to be a Charlie girl. Charlie girls wore Charlie perfume and gold satin jumpsuits and pulled up to restaurants in swanky Rolls Royces. They casually breezed past doormen on their way in and playfully flung their hats at them. A Charlie girl will then move through the crowd like a movie star arriving at the Copacabana while a poorman's Tom Jones sings the Charlie song. *There's a fragrance that's here to stay and they call it—Charlie!* Then a handsome man will grab her and twirl her to their table, when she'll throw her head back with a laugh and settle on the most comely smile ever to say, *Hey there darlin', be a peach and order me a white wine spritzer.*

Charlie girls were happy. They sparkled with optimism and Alberto VO5. You'd certainly never see a Charlie girl pulling up to that restaurant in a beat up old Volkswagen wearing overalls and a baseball cap. And I doubt they would have sold much perfume if you did.

I'm fourteen years old now, looking through a book my brother owns on the Beatles (even though he told me not to) when I come across a photo. And in this photo, John, Paul, George, and Ringo, who are all draped in jewel-toned paisley and floral Indian attire, are sitting cross-legged on the floor with the smiling, bearded Maharishi Mahesh Yogi. This is their guru. There's also a girl for every Beatle, and all four girls have long straight blond hair parted down the middle and are dressed in equally colorful garb with flowers in their hands, and the whole scene looks to me like some kind of psychedelic vortex of freakishly happy hippie folk.

From this photo, I surmise two things:

1. Yoga is from India.

2. Yoga has something to do with LSD.

I'm also under the impression the Beatles were only into yoga because they had already done everything else and they were probably just bored. Also, yoga must have been strictly a sixties thing, seeing how this is 1981-ish and nobody is talking about it. Nor do people dress like they're on the cover of the Sgt. Pepper's album. And by the time *Abbey Road* came out not even the Beatles were dressing like that anymore, so yoga must have been a phase for them.

I'm eighteen. I'm standing on the end of a pier in the middle of the night smoking cloves listening to the guy I'm completely in love with telling me he doesn't think we should see each other anymore.

Men were such assholes.

Two years later, I'm living in an apartment with my friend Jana on the island where we had our summer home. Jana and I had a next-door neighbor whose name I don't remember, but who happened to be one of the first people I ever knew who was sober in AA. I was *not* sober. So one day I got to talking with him and I asked him what it was like, and he said at first it was like being at home and all of a sudden you hear a car screech up onto the driveway, and you look outside where there's a hideous monster behind the wheel of a smoking, backfiring, barely drivable old jalopy, and the monster who is six sizes too big for it is screaming, "HEY YOU UP THERE—GET IN!! GET IN THE CAR!! I KNOW YOU WANT TO, SO JUST GET IN ALREADY AND LET'S GOOOO!!" And after a few years, it's more like being at home, and every once in a while you'll glance out your window, and you'll see a very normal looking guy maybe in a Honda Prelude sitting there, and the guy will say in a very normal voice, "Hey, wanna ride?"

I felt bad for sober people. It sounded like torture. They should've just drunk.

Two years after that, I got sober.

And now I'm twenty-five years old, standing outside Spaghetti Western on Haight Street in San Francisco, where I also lived for about five minutes, probably wearing someone's old confirmation dress from the seventies and black combat boots (because it's 1992 and that's what I always wore). I'm also with my friend Chris, who sees his friend so-and-so who looks exactly like the kind of guy who's either on his way to band practice or maybe an emo poetry reading. Ends up, he says he's on his way to yoga.

I literally remember nothing else about that guy. But I do remember thinking he must have been very lost in life if that's what he felt like he needed.

Me, I was done having problems. That's how you think after you get sober at twenty-two. There's a thought that floats around in the back of your mind: *I've had my struggle. Nothing bad can ever happen to me again, at least not until I'm, like, eighty. Glad I got that out of the way.* You assume you're immune. And it would be pretty unfair if the universe just kept piling problems on you. Come to think of it, there really should be a limit.

Four years later, out of sheer curiosity, I wandered into my first yoga class at the gym in West Hollywood. I had no idea what I was doing and I loved it. The language alone was infatuating: Chaturanga. Rajakapotasana. Vinyasa. I think it was the first time in my life I did something good for myself not because I had to, but because I wanted to.

Twenty years later, I'm still doing yoga.

Right around this time, I was working in a bar with a guy named Rickie. Rickie was French Canadian and super-hot. I adored him. I always thought Rickie and I would have made a great looking couple if he weren't, A) two inches shorter than me, and B) gay.

One night Rickie showed up to work an hour after he found out he was HIV positive. I couldn't believe my eyes. There he was, behind the bar, rarin' to pour Jack and Cokes for people who probably didn't just find out they had a dreaded virus, whose lovers hadn't died of AIDS the year before, and who didn't pay their rent in wads of twenty dollar bills. *And* he seemed totally calm about it. *What the hell was wrong with Rickie?* I didn't want to be around when it hit him.

A month went by. Rickie didn't fall apart. I never even saw him so much as sulk over it. In fact, he ended up telling me being HIV positive was the best thing that had ever happened to him. *What??* At the time, I just couldn't wrap my head around it. *Hi, here's a ticking time bomb for you to hold. Off you go. Be happy.* Frankly, the whole thing terrified the living crap out of me. It could have been anything. And what if I was next? *WHAT IF I WAS NEXT?*

Breaking News: After Receiving a Shocking Diagnosis of (*insert scary disease here), L.A. Woman Throws Herself off Hollywood Sign. Film at 11:00.

Not Rickie. He ate better, slept better. He quit drinking. He took care of himself. I think he may have even done yoga. And he seemed so well adjusted about the whole thing. Happy, even. I admired him for finding the upshot to the situation and all, but there was no way in hell I'd ever understand how you could be truly happy if you had to be *forced* into it.

You see this kind of thing all the time. It used to make me very nervous. *My multimillion-dollar consulting business went belly-up, now I live on a farm raising alpacas and I've never been happier.* I felt like people were settling into their doom awfully easily. They'd reach a certain age and not care that they had to give stuff up. Thirty (casual sex). Forty (cholesterol). Fifty (heels). And they always said the same thing: *I don't care. I'm happy.* It didn't sparkle. It made no sense. They weren't even trying.

You never want to learn your lesson the hard way,

as in the sick or broke or otherwise down-and-out way. No one sits around thinking how awesome it would be to lose everything and have to start over. Or wishing for cancer or the ebola virus or whatever to hurry up and find them already in order to experience a new and improved appreciation for life. I like to choose my *own way* to learn stuff, thanks. And given a choice between having nothing wrong and feeling mediocre or having something wrong and being happy, I know what I would have chosen then. And I know what I'd choose now.

Rumi said, "If you desire healing, let yourself fall ill." You realize what's important. Petty stuff stops bothering you, like when the Internet cuts out for an hour. Or when your husband drinks the last Orange Crush (which he just did). You learn to keep an even keel, even though it may seem half the time like the sky is falling and the anxiety behind it can be so overwhelming and downright dizzying that your walk almost feels more akin to a float, like you're the kid from *The Phantom Tollbooth* whose feet don't actually touch the ground because he grows from the top down. You learn that nothing is the end of the world, not even illness.

This goes for most of the time. Other times I'd like to rip its fucking head right off if it had one.

Fourteen years ago I started working in a different bar with the man I ended up marrying, even though we barely said one word to each other for the first six and a half years. I was "that blonde girl who did yoga" and Mauro was "that Australian dude who worked in the sound booth." One day I made a joke about a dingo eating his baby and then we fell in love.

Sometimes I forget it goes both ways, that amazing things can happen out of the blue just like not-so-amazing things. And how easy it is to miss it all because you're so consumed with worry about other things that usually don't matter. And it may be something that happened last week, or four years ago, or maybe hasn't even happened yet, which is probably the most pointless thing of all for you to worry about, considering that thing *doesn't even exist.* Then there's what *does* exist, and maybe it's something you find so totally unacceptable that all you want to do is resist it or control it or weasel out of it, even though that's what the real problem is and what Buddhists call *dukkha.* AKA suffering. It's dissatisfaction with the world as it is, and the ensuing inability to cope instead of just accepting the fact that not everything is hunky dory all the time, and it never will be. That is just life. And we need to get that through our thick skulls.

"Suffering is not holding you," wrote Osho. "You are holding suffering. When you become good at the art of letting sufferings go, then you'll come to realize how unnecessary it was for you to drag those burdens around with you. You'll see that no one else other than you is responsible. The truth is that existence wants your life to become a festival."

Six years ago I was in a yoga class when my teacher Maria Cristina told this story from the nineteenth-century yoga master Ramakrishna.

Three men are walking in a field. And in the middle of the field, they come to a place surrounded by a high wall. And behind the wall, they can hear the faint sound of instruments playing and people singing. The three guys are dying to know what's on the other side, and sure enough, they see a ladder. So one of the guys starts climbing up it while the other two watch. And when the guy gets to the top and sees what's on the other side, he's beside himself. He can't believe it. He starts uncontrollably laughing and jumps over the wall. Then the second guy climbs up the ladder, and the same exact thing happens. He gets to the top, bursts into laughter and jumps in there too. Then the third guy climbs up the ladder, and when he gets to the top and sees what's going on down there, he can't believe it. It's astonishing. It's the most beautiful thing he's ever seen, because what he's seeing is a raging festival of happiness. People have lost their minds. It's all love and light and beauty down there. It's the happiest sight imaginable. All the guy wants to do is jump down there and join them.

But then he thinks, if I go down there, *nobody else will ever know this place exists.*

So he climbs back down the ladder and tells everyone he can find about the wild, magical sight he had seen and about all the happiness.

Three months later, I find out I have Parkinson's. It's a Monday. The very next day I get the flu. Then that Friday night I leave the house to go to work at the bar and my car is gone.

I text Mauro in a panic, even though he's already at work doing sound checks for some secret show happening that night and he can't help me, telling him "my car got stolen."

He texts me back, "Are you sure? Read the signs."

I read the signs. It turns out I had pulled a bonehead move by parking it in the wrong place and it got towed.

Not my best week.

I'm now running late. So I call my friend Ronna and make her come get me and take me down to the bar, where we see a massive amount of people lined up down the block. And when I walk in the door, I find out the Foo Fighters are playing. I got to watch Dave Grohl and the Foo Fighters play that night from ten feet away, and it was packed in there, and unbelievably loud, and I spent three hours screaming and dancing my head off behind the bar and nothing else mattered. Absolutely nothing. Everything was suddenly okay. The world could have ended and I wouldn't have cared. I'll never forget that feeling.

And that's the scene I picture when I tell the story about the three guys looking over the wall.

It doesn't always sparkle. I don't care anymore. I'm happy.

SUTURED #4: A BRIEF GUIDE THROUGH THE YOGA SUTRAS

BOOK FOUR

PORTION ON ABSOLUTENESS

1. You got the power, babe. It's been in you all along. If you want to blaze up and think about this, go right ahead, yoga's okay with it. Or just do some chanting. And a lot of hard-ass yoga.

2. You can evolve or go back. People do it all the time. This is why there are so many animals.

3. All you're really doing is removing stuff that may be blocking the flow of energy.

4. So don't let that nasty ego tell you who you aren't.

5. Because as many lives as you've led, which may have been millions before you got to be a human, there's only one you.

6. And you don't really want to keep coming back to this whirling rock in the sky to keep trying to get it right. Don't you think this nonsense is getting rather old?

7. People are kind of judging you, which is not cool considering we're all supposed to be in this together. But you do yoga, so you're all, *whatever.*

8. Reminder: Your life is the result of all your past actions. You are your own karma.

9. And regardless of when or where you're born, your karma stays with you.

10. You're stuck with it. Like a Siamese twin.

11. But once you get rid of the cause, it's gone for good. Sayonara, baby!

12. And there goes the difference between the past, present, and future. Because by now they've melted into each other like Salvador Dali clocks and become one.

13. And the awesome thing is you're not resisting it.

14. And remember that pencil we were talking about last time? Depending on the day, you might not see it as a pencil. It could be a stabbing device.

15. So it's the same thing. But not.

16. It also doesn't really matter what you think, because that pencil is going to exist no matter what you call it.

17. And so will a lot of other things. You just don't know it because there's no way you *could* know it. If you can't see infrared light, imagine what else is out there. It's a pretty huge universe.

18. But the *real* you, the one deep down inside, always knows what's up.

19. Although the real you doesn't sit around thinking about how it's the real you.

20. The real you isn't the one that thinks anyway. Your consciousness is the thing that thinks, and as a general rule your consciousness can't think of things and itself at the same time.

21. That would be very confusing. And life is confusing enough.

22. The fact is, the real you never, ever changes. It just has on different skin sometimes.

23. And when you realize this, everything will suddenly make sense.

24. The whole reason bodies exists in the first place is so you have somewhere to live. Otherwise you'd just be floating out there in space.

25. There's a word for understanding this: Freedom.

26. Full on, Age of Aquarius, honey-soaked, hippie-style freedom.

27. You'll get it, because you do yoga. Then you'll lose it. And get it back again. And lose it again. And get it back again.

28. And that is why you have to keep going to yoga forever.

29. But don't go chasing freedom. Don't be calling freedom fifteen times a day and stalking it at work. Big no-no.

30. And don't worry. You're working your ass off here. Karma's bound to wrap itself up one day.

31. And at that point, there's not much else for you to do.

32. Wait—So then are you done?

33. Yup. Hasta la vista, baby.

34. And just like that, it all goes back where it came from. The end.

This is my story. I don't know where I'm going, but I know I'm going somewhere beautiful, and I know I'm on my way. It's been a beautiful adventure. It always will be.

—CHARLOTTE ERIKSSON

TWELVE

RIDE THAT VINYASA

LIKE A HOT BITCH

Let's go. Rev your engines. Pull up to the bumper, baby, and look up.

Spread your fingers wide, there's power there. Stay rooted, reach high, and let the palms touch. There's a heaven above where freedom waits.

Bow down and slide the prayer toward the earth. Ride the yellow Slip 'n Slide down toward a Candy Cane Forest and over Gum Drop Mountain, through a dreamy landscape of every memory and every misstep you've ever made along the way until now.

I know what I'd see: a black-and-white wedding photo, my parents, 1959. A Ferris wheel, a puka shell necklace, the prism on the cover of *The Dark Side of the Moon*. A seaside arcade. A stack of old notebooks—my first attempts at writing. My past in one-hundred-page increments.

Lift halfway up. Flat back. Offer the heart. Take a moment in between breaths to let yourself see what's left to be seen, all the places you've been. Your old haunts. I pass by them every day, and after all these years I'll find myself wondering if they're just facades, like the saloon fronts and gun shops of an old ghost town set. As if I can poke my head inside the doors in the light of day and see nothing but framed out rooms and sandy floors, existing for no other reason than to give structure to who I used to be.

Two things there will always be in life: beauty and pain. Mostly beauty.

Step back from here and pause. You're stronger than you think, strong as a plank of wood. Bend your elbows and keep it steady as you lower down toward the ground in the shape of the four-pointed staff, and let yourself hover.

This is all there is.

This is your life.

It might break your heart, like an aria. And it can sting, like a slap in the temple. But think about your beautiful world, of all that you've been given, all that's been taken, and all that's left until you've got nowhere to look but up, like the earthy Black Mamba. Deadly, like venom. And lovely, like reincarnation.

Who knows the meaning of life and death, or anything else quasi-important. Maybe the starving poets on street corners and oceanside piers. I'd give 'em my last dollar to inspire me. That's all I really want.

Now move over, Rover, and take it slowly up and back. You're facing downward now, on the joyride of your life. Crank the music and take it all the way down Sunset Boulevard, through Hollywood to the epic ocean, when you've apparently reached the end of the Earth. Sing out loud and let yourself be free. And remember what Johnny Cash once said of the songs that helped bring him back from the despair of his addictions: "At times they've been my only way back, the only door out of the dark, bad places the black dog calls home."

Take a brave step forward. You can do it. We'll make it together. Rise up and lift your sword, peaceful warrior. Keep it strong and steady. You've already lived and fought a thousand battles, and you're not here—*again*—to cower in fear and pain. Love without conflict, fight for it without malice, and keep an open heart. Everything you've been through will be worth it.

And life will ebb and flow, a little easier, like water. And sweeter now, like honey.

NOTES

77 *"To remain stable is to refrain from"*: Alan Watts, *The Wisdom of Insecurity: A Message for an Age of Anxiety*, Vintage Books, 2011.

162 *"The Now is as it is"*: Eckhart Tolle, *Stillness Speaks*, Namaste Publishing and New World Library, 2010.

169 *"all one can do is hope"*: Arthur Miller, *The Ride Down Mount Morgan*, Stage & Screen, 1991.

186 *"The most beautiful thing we can experience"*: Albert Einstein, *Living Philosophies*, Simon and Schuster, 1931.

199 *"The life of every man is a diary"*: J. M. Barrie, *The Little Minister*, Echo Library, 2007.

219 *"Life is a series of natural and spontaneous changes"*: Lao Tzu, from *1001 Pearls of Spiritual Wisdom*, edited by Kim Lim, Skyhorse Publishing, 2015.

246 *"At times they've been my only way back"*: Johnny Cash, *Cash: The Autobiography*, HarperSanFrancisco, 1997, 29.

ACKNOWLEDGMENTS

Thank you to everyone who encouraged and supported me during the writing of this book.

Thank you John Clendening, the most amazing big brother in the history of brothers. I only hope one day I can write as beautifully as you. Love, Tater.

Thank you Ronna Holtz. You have the most open heart of anyone I know. Never change. And never throw away the sweatshirt with the dancing skeleton.

Thank you Jalee Carder. If I ever win the lottery I will buy the house next door for you and Gia so we can grow old together and reminisce about our Hollywood heydays. It'll be kind of like now, but with a pool.

Thank you Christina Natale. Who knew we'd be here almost twenty-five years after we bonded over broken sugar cookies. You are a truly loyal friend.

Thank you Solana Mejia. My little sister. And the one

person who will sit here with me all day and watch seven horror movies in a row. And maybe a few bad ones.

Thank you Catia Salvadori. You are way too far away these days, but only because your life is so big and beautiful it had no other choice to expand all the way to Nashville. No one deserves it more than you.

Thank you Gretchen Westlake. Pilot to co-pilot. We'll always have each other.

Thank you Debra Ollivier. Your confidence in me has meant everything.

Thank you Onorina Rubbi for being a second mother to me. And to my father-in-law Mario for calling me his "piccolo amore."

Finally, thank you to my husband Mauro. My favorite person in the world. I love you.

RELATED TITLES

Awake at 3:00 a.m.
SUZANNAH NEUFELD

Holding Space
AMY WRIGHT GLENN

No Mud, No Lotus
THICH NHAT HANH

Ocean of Insight
HEATHER LYN MANN

Strange Beauty
ELIZA FACTOR